The Late-Diagnosed Autism Career Handbook

From Discovery to Professional Success

I0039024

Arabela Susie Raymond

Copyright © 2025 by Arabela Susie Raymond

All rights reserved. No part of this publication may be reproduced, distributed, or transmitted in any form or by any means, including photocopying, recording, or other electronic or mechanical methods, without the prior written permission of the publisher, except in the case of brief quotations embodied in critical reviews and certain other noncommercial uses permitted by copyright law.

This book is designed to provide information and motivation to readers. It is sold with the understanding that the publisher and author are not engaged in rendering any type of psychological, legal, medical, or any other kind of professional advice. The content is the sole expression and opinion of the author and not necessarily that of the publisher. No warranties or guarantees are expressed or implied by the choice to include any of the content in this book. The author and publisher shall have neither liability nor responsibility to any person or entity with respect to any loss or damage caused, or alleged to have been caused, directly or indirectly, by the information provided in this book.

The strategies outlined in this book may not be suitable for every situation. This work is sold with the understanding that the author and publisher are not held responsible for the results accruing from the advice in this book.

Names and scenarios depicted in this book are purely for illustrative purposes only. Any resemblance to actual persons, living or dead, or actual events is purely coincidental.

The advice and strategies found within may not be suitable for every situation. This work is sold with the understanding that neither the author nor the publisher are held responsible for the results accruing from the advice in this book.

ISBN: 978-1-7641438-6-8

Isohan Publishing

Table of Contents

Preface

The conference room was silent except for the hum of fluorescent lights and the soft clicking of keyboards. Sarah, a 37-year-old operations director, sat reviewing her quarterly presentation when her phone buzzed with a message from her therapist: "Your autism assessment results are ready." Three months later, that same conference room felt completely different—not because anything had changed in the environment, but because Sarah finally understood why she processed information systematically, why small talk drained her energy, and why her attention to detail had made her indispensable to her organization.

Sarah's story isn't unique. Across industries and career levels, professionals are receiving autism diagnoses in their thirties, forties, and beyond, fundamentally reframing their understanding of workplace challenges they've navigated for decades. This handbook emerges from the recognition that late-diagnosed autistic professionals face a unique set of circumstances that existing career resources don't address.

Why This Book Exists

When I began researching autism workplace success, I discovered a troubling gap. Most career guidance assumes either childhood diagnosis with supported transition to employment, or focuses on entry-level job acquisition. Virtually nothing existed for professionals who've built careers, earned promotions, and established expertise— only to discover that their brain works differently than they'd always assumed.

Late-diagnosed autistic professionals aren't starting from scratch. They're recontextualizing years or decades of work experience through a new lens of self-understanding. They need strategies that build on existing career momentum while addressing challenges they now recognize as autism-related rather than personal inadequacies.

This handbook fills that gap by providing career advancement strategies specifically designed for the late-diagnosed autism experience.

How This Book Works: The Power of Recognition

Each chapter in this handbook begins with a detailed case study featuring a late-diagnosed autistic professional navigating specific workplace challenges. These aren't generic examples—they're carefully constructed scenarios that reflect real patterns I've observed in the autism professional community.

I chose this case study approach because recognition drives transformation. When you see your own experience reflected in someone else's story, several powerful things happen simultaneously: you realize you're not alone in facing these challenges, you understand that your struggles aren't personal failings, and you begin to see patterns that point toward solutions.

Consider how Sarah's story might have resonated with you. Perhaps you recognized the systematic information processing, the energy drain from social performance, or the way environments feel different once you understand your sensory needs. This recognition creates the emotional foundation necessary for implementing practical career strategies.

The Clinical Practice Approach

My writing style deliberately mirrors clinical practice methodology—clear, systematic, and focused on actionable outcomes. Each chapter follows a structured format: case study recognition, pattern analysis, evidence-based strategies, and practical implementation tools. This approach serves autism readers particularly well because it provides the logical structure and detailed guidance that support autism learning styles.

The case studies serve multiple functions beyond simple illustration. They demonstrate how autism traits appear in professional settings, show the thought processes that lead to effective solutions, and provide models for applying strategies in your own career situations. Rather than abstract advice, you'll see exactly how professionals like yourself have navigated similar challenges successfully.

Real People, Real Solutions

Every case study in this handbook represents composite experiences drawn from interviews with late-diagnosed autistic professionals across industries and career levels. While names and specific details are fictional, the challenges, thought processes, and solutions reflect real experiences of real people who've transformed their careers through autism-informed strategies.

The scenarios progress from immediate workplace challenges through long-term career development, mirroring the journey most late-diagnosed professionals experience. You'll recognize your own story in these pages, but you'll also see possibilities for your future that you might not have considered.

How to Use This Handbook

This handbook functions as both a complete career development system and a reference resource for specific challenges. You can read it sequentially for comprehensive career planning, or access individual chapters for targeted solutions to immediate workplace issues.

Each chapter includes practical action items that translate concepts into concrete steps you can implement immediately. Templates, worksheets, and protocols provide tools you can adapt to your specific situation and communication style.

The appendices offer additional resources including industry-specific considerations, emergency protocols for workplace crises, and comprehensive references for ongoing professional development.

Your Professional Renaissance Begins

Your autism diagnosis represents the beginning of your professional renaissance—a period of renewed growth based on authentic self-understanding rather than neurotypical performance. The strategies in this handbook will help you leverage your systematic thinking, analytical capabilities, and attention to detail as professional strengths while managing the environmental and social challenges that may have limited your career satisfaction.

The professionals whose stories fill these pages have built successful careers not despite their autism, but because they learned to work with their autistic brains rather than against them. Their experiences provide the roadmap for your own career transformation.

Your journey from discovery to professional success starts here, with recognition that your autism isn't something to overcome—it's your foundation for authentic career excellence.

Introduction

Your Career Rediscovered

The phone call came on a Tuesday afternoon. Sarah, a 38-year-old marketing director, sat in her car after another exhausting day at the office, staring at the autism assessment report she'd just received. The words "Autism Spectrum Disorder" felt foreign yet oddly familiar. After decades of feeling different, struggling with office politics, and wondering why networking events left her drained for days, she finally had an answer.

You might recognize yourself in Sarah's story. Maybe you've recently received your own diagnosis, or perhaps you're still wondering if autism explains those workplace patterns you've never quite understood. The late diagnosis of autism doesn't just change how you see yourself—it transforms everything about how you approach your professional life.

Welcome to Your Professional Renaissance

This moment marks the beginning of your professional renaissance. The diagnosis you've received isn't an ending or a limitation—it's the key that unlocks decades of confusion about your work life. Every job that felt impossible, every workplace interaction that seemed unnecessarily complex, every time you went home exhausted after what others called "just another day at the office" now makes sense.

Consider Marcus, a 42-year-old software engineer who spent fifteen years believing he was simply "bad at teamwork." His autism diagnosis revealed that his preference for written communication over spontaneous meetings wasn't a character flaw—it was how his brain processed information most effectively. Once he understood this, he could advocate for communication methods that actually worked, transforming both his productivity and job satisfaction.

The late diagnosis experience differs significantly from childhood diagnosis. You've built a career, developed coping mechanisms, and created professional relationships—all while navigating the world without understanding your neurological differences. This foundation becomes your strength, not your burden.

Why Late Diagnosis Changes Everything About Work

Your autism diagnosis reframes your entire professional narrative. Those "personality quirks" that made certain jobs unbearable suddenly make perfect sense. The sensory overload from open offices, the confusion during ambiguous instructions, the exhaustion from constant social performance—these weren't personal failings but predictable responses to environments that didn't match your neurological needs.

Take Jennifer, a 34-year-old financial analyst who thought she lacked ambition because she consistently turned down promotions to management roles. Her autism diagnosis revealed that she instinctively understood management positions would require social and executive function skills that would drain her energy. Her preference for detailed analytical work wasn't career limitation—it was career wisdom.

The diagnosis also illuminates your professional strengths. Your attention to detail isn't obsessiveness—it's quality control. Your need for clear processes isn't rigidity—it's systematic thinking. Your direct communication style isn't rudeness—it's efficiency. These reframes shift you from defending your differences to leveraging your advantages.

Many late-diagnosed professionals report feeling like they've been playing a game without knowing the rules. The diagnosis provides the rulebook. You can stop trying to fit neurotypical expectations and start building a career that works with your brain, not against it.

How to Use This Guide for Immediate and Long-Term Success

This guide operates on two levels: immediate relief and strategic transformation. You need practical solutions for Monday morning's challenges, but you also need a framework for long-term career satisfaction.

Start with your most pressing workplace issues. If sensory overload in your open office is creating daily misery, jump to the environmental modification strategies. If you're considering disclosure to your supervisor, review the decision-making framework first. This isn't a book you must read sequentially—it's a resource you can access based on your current needs.

For immediate implementation, each section includes specific action items. These aren't theoretical exercises but practical tools developed by and for autistic professionals. The accommodation request templates come from successful workplace conversations. The energy management strategies reflect real solutions that prevent burnout.

The long-term transformation requires patience with yourself. You're not just learning new workplace strategies—you're rebuilding your professional identity around authentic self-understanding. This process takes time, and setbacks are normal parts of growth.

David, a 45-year-old project manager, describes his post-diagnosis career journey as "learning to work with my brain instead of fighting it." His first year involved small adjustments—noise-canceling headphones, written meeting summaries, structured check-ins with his team. By year two, he was redesigning project workflows to leverage systematic thinking. By year three, he was training other managers on clear communication practices.

Setting Realistic Expectations for Your Career Transformation

Career transformation after late autism diagnosis isn't about becoming a different person—it's about becoming more authentically yourself in professional settings. This distinction matters because it sets appropriate expectations for change.

Some changes happen quickly. Once you understand your sensory needs, you can modify your workspace within weeks. Accommodation requests, when properly framed, often receive approval faster than expected. Communication strategies can improve workplace relationships almost immediately.

Other changes require longer timelines. Building authentic professional relationships takes time, especially if you've spent years masking your true personality. Career transitions—moving to autism-friendly industries or roles—often require months or years of planning. Developing leadership skills that work with autistic strengths involves ongoing practice and refinement.

The transformation also isn't linear. You'll have days when everything clicks and you wonder why work ever felt difficult. You'll have other days when old patterns resurface and you question your progress. Both experiences are normal parts of integrating your diagnosis into your professional life.

Realistic expectations also mean accepting that not every workplace will be autism-friendly, regardless of legal requirements. Some organizational cultures remain hostile to neurological differences. Part of your career strategy involves identifying environments where you can thrive and avoiding those where you'll struggle unnecessarily.

Lisa, a 41-year-old human resources director, spent her first post-diagnosis year trying to make her current role work through accommodations and communication improvements. When these efforts yielded minimal change, she realized the problem wasn't her approach but her environment. Her transition to a smaller, more structured organization transformed her work experience entirely.

Your career transformation also affects others in your life. Family members might need time to understand how your diagnosis changes your work needs. Colleagues might adjust to new communication preferences or workspace modifications. These relationship adjustments require patience and clear explanation.

The most realistic expectation is that this guide provides tools, not guarantees. Every workplace is different, every autistic person is unique, and every career path presents distinct challenges. What works for one person might not work for another. Your job is to experiment with different strategies, adapt them to your situation, and build a personalized approach to professional success.

Success looks different for different people. For some, success means thriving in their current role with new self-awareness and accommodations. For others, success requires complete career changes to autism-friendly fields. Some find success in traditional employment, while others create alternative career paths through consulting or entrepreneurship.

The common thread among successful late-diagnosed autistic professionals isn't any specific career choice—it's the willingness to honor their authentic selves in professional settings. They stop trying to be neurotypical and start optimizing for their actual strengths and needs.

Your diagnosis doesn't limit your career potential—it clarifies your path to professional fulfillment. The strategies in this guide help you navigate that path with confidence, authenticity, and sustainable success.

Key Insights to Remember

- Your autism diagnosis reframes workplace challenges as neurological differences, not personal failures
- Professional transformation happens at both immediate and strategic levels

- Change timelines vary from immediate environmental modifications to long-term career transitions

- Success means building a career that works with your autistic brain, not against it

- Every autistic professional's path looks different, but authenticity remains the common success factor

The journey ahead combines practical problem-solving with identity integration. You're not just changing how you work—you're discovering who you are as an autistic professional. This discovery process, while sometimes challenging, leads to career satisfaction that many neurotypical professionals never experience.

Your next chapter begins with understanding exactly how autism shows up in professional settings and why this understanding changes everything about workplace success.

Chapter 1: Reframing Your Career Story Through an Autism Lens

The conference room felt different that Thursday morning. Not because anything had changed in the sterile corporate environment where Rachel had worked for twelve years—same fluorescent lights, same uncomfortable chairs, same colleagues discussing quarterly projections. But Rachel herself had changed. Three weeks after receiving her autism diagnosis at age 39, she finally understood why her career had felt like a series of puzzles with missing pieces.

You're about to experience this same shift in perspective. Your autism diagnosis doesn't just explain workplace difficulties—it reveals patterns in your professional life that suddenly make perfect sense. The jobs that felt impossible weren't failures; they were mismatches. The roles where you thrived weren't accidents; they were environments that naturally supported your autistic brain.

Recognizing Patterns You Never Understood Before

Your career story contains patterns that have been hiding in plain sight. Once you understand autism, these patterns become clear roadmaps showing exactly why certain professional experiences felt easy while others felt insurmountable.

Start with the jobs that made you question your competence. Maybe you struggled in a customer service role that required constant social interaction and unpredictable problem-solving. Or perhaps a project management position that demanded juggling multiple priorities left you feeling overwhelmed and ineffective. These weren't character flaws—they were predictable responses to environments that didn't match your neurological processing style.

Consider Tom, a 44-year-old engineer who spent five years in business development, consistently missing sales targets despite technical expertise that impressed clients. His autism diagnosis revealed that the open-ended networking requirements and unpredictable client interactions created constant sensory and social overload. His perceived sales inadequacy was actually his brain protecting itself from overwhelming stimulation.

The pattern recognition extends beyond obvious struggles. You might notice that positions requiring detailed analysis, systematic processes, or independent work felt naturally comfortable. These weren't just personality preferences—they were your brain operating in its optimal mode.

Review your performance evaluations over the years. Look for repeated themes about communication style, team collaboration, or attention to detail. Comments about being "too direct" or "overly focused on minor issues" often reflect autism traits that supervisors didn't understand. Positive feedback about reliability, thoroughness, or innovative thinking highlights your autistic strengths in action.

Many late-diagnosed professionals describe feeling like they were "faking it" in certain roles. This feeling makes sense now—you were working against your natural processing style, requiring enormous energy to maintain performance that came easily to neurotypical colleagues.

Why Certain Jobs Felt Impossible While Others Energized You

The difference between draining and energizing work experiences relates directly to how well the job environment matched your autistic brain's needs. Jobs that felt impossible typically violated multiple autism-friendly principles, while energizing roles naturally supported your neurological differences.

Impossible jobs often shared common characteristics. They required constant social interaction without recovery time. They demanded rapid task-switching between unrelated projects. They operated in chaotic environments with unpredictable schedules and unclear expectations. They emphasized networking and relationship-building over technical competence.

Sarah, a 41-year-old marketing professional, describes her previous role in event planning as "three years of daily torture." The constant vendor negotiations, last-minute changes, and high-pressure social events created perfect conditions for autism burnout. She blamed herself for lacking "people skills" until her diagnosis revealed that the role's demands directly conflicted with her need for structure and predictability.

Energizing jobs typically provided structure, clear expectations, and opportunities to use your natural strengths. They allowed focused work time without constant interruptions. They valued quality over quantity and provided feedback based on concrete results rather than subjective social performance.

Marcus, a 38-year-old data analyst, found his current role "accidentally perfect" for his autistic brain. The work requires deep focus on complex datasets, follows systematic analytical processes, and produces clear, measurable outcomes. His manager values his thorough reports and rarely requires spontaneous meetings. What Marcus initially saw as career luck was actually an environment that naturally supported his autism traits.

The energy difference between these job types reflects the metabolic cost of masking. Impossible jobs required constant masking—suppressing your natural responses, forcing social performance, and maintaining neurotypical facades. This masking consumed enormous mental energy, leaving you exhausted and questioning your professional capabilities.

Energizing jobs allowed more authentic self-expression. You could communicate directly, work systematically, and focus on tasks rather than social performance. The energy you previously spent on masking became available for actual work, improving both your performance and job satisfaction.

Identifying Your Unrecognized Autistic Strengths in Past Roles

Your career history contains numerous examples of autistic strengths that were never properly recognized or labeled. These strengths appeared as exceptional performance in specific areas, often dismissed as "just being detail-oriented" or "naturally analytical."

Systematic problem-solving shows up in roles where you consistently identified root causes that others missed. You approached problems methodically, considered multiple variables, and developed solutions that addressed underlying issues rather than surface symptoms. Colleagues might have called this "overthinking," but it was actually thorough analysis.

Jennifer, a 35-year-old operations manager, consistently prevented manufacturing errors by creating detailed process documentation that others considered excessive. Her autism diagnosis revealed that her need for clarity and structure naturally produced quality control systems that saved her company hundreds of thousands of dollars in defects and recalls.

Pattern recognition appeared in your ability to spot trends, predict outcomes, or identify connections that weren't obvious to others. This strength often manifested in strategic planning, data analysis, or process improvement initiatives. You saw patterns because your brain naturally processes information systematically.

Attention to detail went beyond simple carefulness. You caught errors others missed, maintained quality standards even under pressure, and produced work that consistently met high standards. This wasn't perfectionism—it was your brain's natural tendency toward thoroughness and accuracy.

Consistent performance meant you delivered reliable results regardless of external circumstances. While others' performance fluctuated based on mood, politics, or motivation, your systematic approach produced steady, predictable outcomes. This reliability made you trusted for important projects even when colleagues didn't understand your working style.

Innovation through different perspectives showed up as solutions that others hadn't considered. Your autism brain approaches problems differently, often finding creative solutions by following logical paths that neurotypical thinkers miss. These innovations might have been labeled as "thinking outside the box," but they were actually systematic thinking applied to complex problems.

Review your career achievements through this lens. Projects you managed successfully, problems you solved uniquely, and processes you improved all likely reflect autistic strengths in action. These weren't accidental successes—they were your brain operating at its best.

Common Career Trajectories of Late-Diagnosed Professionals

Late-diagnosed autistic professionals often follow predictable career patterns that reflect their attempts to find neurologically compatible work environments. Understanding these patterns helps you recognize your own journey and plan more intentional career moves.

The False Start Pattern involves initial career choices that seemed logical but proved unsustainable. You might have chosen careers based on external expectations, salary potential, or social prestige rather than neurological fit. These early roles often ended in burnout, job changes, or career pivots that felt like failures at the time.

David started his career in pharmaceutical sales, attracted by the technical training and product knowledge requirements. However, the constant cold calling, relationship management, and quota pressure created chronic stress that led to anxiety and depression. He eventually transitioned to medical writing, where his scientific knowledge and attention to detail made him exceptionally successful. His "failed" sales career was actually valuable data about his autism needs.

The Accidental Success Pattern describes finding career satisfaction through trial and error rather than intentional planning. You stumbled into roles that worked well for your autistic brain, often without understanding why these positions felt different from previous jobs.

Lisa discovered technical writing after being laid off from a marketing coordinator role. The structured writing process, clear deadlines, and minimal social interaction created an environment where her autism traits became professional assets. She thought she was lucky to find work she enjoyed—actually, she had found autism-compatible employment.

The Specialist Trajectory involves developing deep expertise in specific areas rather than broad generalist skills. You built careers around technical competencies, detailed knowledge, or specialized skills that leveraged your autistic strengths.

Michael became a database administrator after struggling in general IT support roles. His systematic approach to data management and ability to focus on complex problems for extended periods made him exceptionally skilled at database optimization and security. His career success came from playing to autism strengths rather than fighting autism challenges.

The Entrepreneurial Escape describes leaving traditional employment to create autism-friendly work environments.

This pattern often emerges after years of workplace struggles, leading to consulting, freelancing, or business ownership that allows control over work conditions.

Anna left corporate accounting to start her own bookkeeping service after realizing that her need for quiet work spaces and detailed processes conflicted with modern open-office environments. Her business success came from creating work conditions that supported rather than hindered her autistic brain.

Action Items: Career Pattern Mapping Exercise

Complete this systematic analysis of your career patterns to identify autism-related themes and plan future moves.

Step 1: Career Timeline Creation List every job you've held for more than six months, including:

- Job title and industry
- Duration of employment
- Reason for leaving
- Energy level during the role (1-10 scale)
- Notable achievements or struggles

Step 2: Pattern Identification Review your timeline and identify:

- Jobs that felt energizing vs. draining
- Common characteristics of successful roles
- Repeated challenges across different positions
- Moments of exceptional performance or recognition

- Times when you felt like you were "faking it"

Step 3: Autism Lens Analysis For each position, evaluate:

- **Sensory environment**: Was the workspace comfortable or overwhelming?

- **Social demands**: How much interpersonal interaction was required?

- **Structure level**: Were expectations clear or ambiguous?

- **Task variety**: Did you focus on specific areas or juggle multiple priorities?

- **Communication style**: Could you communicate directly or was diplomacy required?

Step 4: Strength Recognition Identify instances where autism traits appeared as professional strengths:

- Systematic problem-solving that others missed

- Pattern recognition that provided valuable insights

- Attention to detail that prevented errors or improved quality

- Consistent performance during challenging periods

- Innovation through different thinking approaches

Step 5: Future Planning Framework Based on your pattern analysis, create guidelines for future career decisions:

- Environmental requirements for optimal performance

- Types of tasks that energize vs. drain you

- Communication and social interaction preferences

- Industries or roles that typically support autism traits
- Red flags to avoid in job searches or career moves

This analysis provides concrete data about your autism-related career patterns, moving you from intuitive job selection to strategic career planning based on neurological compatibility.

Moving Forward with Clarity

Your career story hasn't been a series of random events or personal failures. It's been a journey toward understanding how your autistic brain functions in professional environments. Every job that felt impossible taught you something about your needs. Every role that energized you revealed something about your strengths.

This reframing doesn't minimize past struggles—it provides context that transforms those struggles from personal inadequacies into data about neurological fit. You weren't failing at those difficult jobs; you were working against your brain's natural processing style while lacking the self-awareness to make informed career choices.

The career pattern mapping exercise provides the foundation for all future professional decisions. You now have concrete data about what works, what doesn't, and why. This knowledge becomes your career compass, guiding you toward opportunities that support rather than hinder your autistic strengths.

Core Insights for Professional Success

- Your career struggles weren't personal failures but predictable responses to autism-incompatible environments

- Jobs that felt energizing naturally supported your neurological processing style

- Autism traits appeared as professional strengths throughout your career, even when not recognized as such

- Late-diagnosed professionals follow common career patterns that reflect unconscious attempts to find neurological compatibility

- Systematic analysis of your career history provides clear guidelines for future professional decisions

Understanding your career through an autism lens transforms confusion into clarity and past struggles into future wisdom. You're ready to build on this foundation by examining the hidden costs of professional masking and learning how to reduce that exhausting performance.

Chapter 2: The Hidden Cost of Professional Masking

The 6:30 PM elevator ride down thirty-seven floors gave Amanda exactly two minutes and fifteen seconds to decompress. Every workday for the past eight years, she used this brief window to let her shoulders drop, stop forcing eye contact, and allow her face to relax from its carefully maintained professional expression. By the time the elevator doors opened in the lobby, she had to be "on" again for the brief social interactions required to exit the building.

This ritual made perfect sense after her autism diagnosis at age 36. She'd been performing neurotypicality for eight hours daily, and that performance had an energy cost she'd never calculated. You've likely paid this same hidden cost throughout your career—masking your autistic traits to meet workplace expectations while never understanding why you felt so drained.

What Workplace Masking Looks Like for Professionals

Professional masking involves suppressing your natural autistic responses and replacing them with learned neurotypical behaviors. Unlike the obvious masking that children might do, professional masking is sophisticated, subtle, and often invisible even to yourself.

Forced eye contact during meetings, presentations, and conversations requires conscious effort and constant monitoring. You've learned to look at foreheads, noses, or just past someone's ear to create the appearance of direct eye contact. This performance demands continuous attention that could otherwise focus on conversation content or meeting objectives.

Scripted social interactions replace natural communication patterns. You've memorized appropriate responses for workplace small talk, learned to ask about weekends and holidays, and developed a repertoire of socially acceptable comments about weather, sports, or current events. These scripts require mental energy to remember, select, and deliver convincingly.

Suppressing stimming behaviors means controlling natural self-regulation mechanisms that help you process sensory input and manage stress. You've learned to keep your hands still during meetings, avoid rocking or swaying, and resist the urge to fidget with objects. This suppression removes your natural coping mechanisms while adding the stress of behavioral monitoring.

Emotional regulation performance involves displaying expected emotional responses rather than authentic ones. You've learned to appear enthusiastic about projects that bore you, concerned about issues that don't affect you, and disappointed by setbacks that you view as learning opportunities. This emotional performance requires constant calibration to match workplace norms.

Consider Robert, a 42-year-old project manager who spent fifteen years believing he was naturally extroverted because he could "work the room" at professional events. His autism diagnosis revealed that his networking ability came from carefully studied social scripts, not innate social skills. He could perform extroversion convincingly, but the energy cost left him exhausted for days after each event.

Cognitive masking involves presenting your thinking process in neurotypical formats rather than your natural systematic approach. You've learned to provide quick answers even when you need processing time, to focus on big-picture summaries rather than detailed analysis, and to participate in brainstorming sessions that feel chaotic and unproductive.

Sensory suppression means ignoring or hiding your responses to uncomfortable environmental stimuli. You've trained yourself not to react visibly to fluorescent lights, open office noise, strong perfumes, or uncomfortable seating. This suppression doesn't eliminate the sensory impact—it just hides your response while the stimulation continues affecting your nervous system.

The Energy Drain of Performing Neurotypicality at Work

Professional masking consumes cognitive resources that could otherwise contribute to work performance, creativity, and job satisfaction. This energy drain operates like a background program running constantly on your mental computer, slowing down all other processes.

Attention splitting occurs when part of your cognitive capacity constantly monitors your behavior, appearance, and social performance. Instead of focusing entirely on work tasks, you're simultaneously managing your professional persona. This divided attention reduces both the quality and efficiency of your actual work output.

Decision fatigue accelerates throughout the day as masking requires thousands of micro-decisions about appropriate responses, expressions, and behaviors. Each interaction demands choices about eye contact duration, facial expressions, vocal tone, and body language. By afternoon, this decision-making burden significantly impacts your capacity for work-related choices.

Maria, a 39-year-old software developer, described her masking fatigue as "running a social simulation program that uses 30% of my processing power all day." She realized that her afternoon productivity decline wasn't due to natural circadian rhythms but to the accumulating energy cost of maintaining her professional mask.

Stress hormone elevation results from the constant vigilance required for successful masking. Your nervous system interprets the continuous monitoring and performance as potential threat situations, maintaining elevated cortisol and adrenaline levels throughout the workday. This chronic stress response contributes to physical symptoms including headaches, muscle tension, and digestive issues.

Executive function depletion occurs as masking demands use the same cognitive resources required for planning, organization, and impulse control. As your masking energy depletes throughout the day, your ability to manage complex tasks, resist distractions, and maintain focus diminishes accordingly.

Reduced creativity and innovation happen when cognitive resources focus on performance rather than problem-solving. Your brain's natural pattern recognition and systematic thinking abilities—key autism strengths—become less available when mental energy goes toward maintaining neurotypical behavior.

Why You've Been Chronically Exhausted After Work

The exhaustion you've experienced after work isn't normal tiredness from productive labor—it's the specific fatigue that comes from sustained masking performance. This exhaustion has distinct characteristics that differ from standard work-related tiredness.

Cognitive overload symptoms include difficulty processing information, making decisions, or engaging in complex thinking after work. You might find yourself unable to follow television shows, read books, or engage in conversations that require mental effort. This isn't laziness; it's cognitive resource depletion from constant masking.

Sensory overwhelm becomes more pronounced after extended masking periods. Sounds seem louder, lights appear brighter, and textures feel more intense. Your suppressed sensory responses throughout the day create a backlog of stimulation that demands processing once you stop masking.

Social withdrawal serves as necessary recovery time rather than antisocial behavior. You need solitude to process the day's social interactions, decompress from performance pressure, and restore your authentic self-expression. This withdrawal isn't unfriendliness—it's neurological recovery.

Kevin, a 40-year-old marketing director, realized that his evening routine of sitting in his car for twenty minutes before going inside wasn't procrastination but necessary decompression time. After masking for nine hours, he needed space to transition from his professional persona back to his authentic self.

Emotional numbing occurs when the energy required for emotional regulation performance throughout the day depletes your capacity for genuine emotional experience. You might feel disconnected from your own feelings, unable to access joy or satisfaction even after professional successes.

Physical symptoms including headaches, muscle tension, and fatigue reflect the physiological cost of sustained stress response. Your body maintains fight-or-flight readiness during masking, leading to physical exhaustion that rest alone doesn't resolve.

Identifying Your Specific Masking Behaviors

Each autistic professional develops unique masking patterns based on their specific traits, work environment, and career requirements. Identifying your personal masking behaviors is essential for developing strategies to reduce their energy cost.

Social masking behaviors might include:

- Forcing participation in office social events or casual conversations

- Laughing at jokes you don't find funny or understand

- Asking questions about topics that don't interest you

- Pretending to enjoy group activities or team-building exercises

- Suppressing your natural communication directness

Sensory masking behaviors often involve:

- Tolerating uncomfortable lighting, noise, or temperature without complaint

- Avoiding fidgeting or self-stimming behaviors in public spaces

- Suppressing visible reactions to strong smells or textures

- Forcing yourself to eat in noisy cafeterias or restaurants

- Enduring open office environments without seeking modifications

Cognitive masking behaviors include:

- Providing immediate responses when you need processing time

- Participating in brainstorming sessions that feel chaotic

- Focusing on big-picture discussions when you prefer details

- Suppressing your natural systematic approach to problems

- Avoiding detailed questions that showcase your depth of knowledge

Emotional masking behaviors encompass:

- Displaying enthusiasm for projects that don't engage you

- Suppressing frustration with illogical processes or decisions

- Performing concern for issues that don't affect you directly

- Hiding your genuine interests and passions
- Moderating your authentic emotional responses to workplace events

Action Items: Masking Audit and Energy Tracking

This systematic approach helps you identify specific masking behaviors and their energy costs, providing data for strategic reduction strategies.

Week 1: Masking Behavior Documentation For five workdays, track your masking behaviors using these categories:

1. **Morning Masking (7-11 AM)**
   - Record specific behaviors you perform to appear neurotypical
   - Note the energy cost on a 1-5 scale for each behavior
   - Identify triggers that prompt masking responses

2. **Midday Masking (11 AM-3 PM)**
   - Document social interactions requiring performance
   - Track sensory suppression and accommodation behaviors
   - Note cognitive masking during meetings or collaborative work

3. **Afternoon Masking (3-7 PM)**
   - Record masking behaviors as energy depletes

- Note increased effort required for same behaviors
- Track any masking failures or slip-ups

Week 2: Energy Impact Analysis Monitor the relationship between masking and energy levels:

1. **Hourly Energy Ratings** Rate your energy level hourly on a 1-10 scale, noting:

    - Energy at start of workday
    - Energy after high-masking activities (meetings, presentations, social interactions)
    - Energy during low-masking periods (independent work, email)
    - End-of-day energy levels

2. **Recovery Time Tracking** Document recovery requirements:

    - Time needed to decompress after work
    - Activities that help restore energy
    - Days when recovery extends into evening or weekend

3. **Performance Correlation** Note connections between masking intensity and work quality:

    - Tasks that suffer when masking energy is high
    - Work quality during low-masking periods
    - Creativity and problem-solving effectiveness relative to masking demands

Week 3: Pattern Recognition Analyze your two weeks of data to identify:

1. **Highest-cost masking behaviors**
   - Which performances require the most energy
   - Times of day when masking becomes most difficult
   - Specific work situations that demand intensive masking

2. **Natural masking breaks**
   - Work activities that allow authentic self-expression
   - Colleagues who require minimal masking
   - Physical spaces or times that support authenticity

3. **Masking optimization opportunities**
   - Behaviors that could be modified rather than eliminated
   - Situations where reduced masking might be acceptable
   - Environmental changes that could reduce masking demands

Implementation Planning Based on your analysis, develop strategies for:

- Reducing high-cost masking behaviors through environmental modifications

- Scheduling recovery time throughout the workday

- Communicating needs in ways that reduce masking requirements

- Building authentic relationships that support reduced performance

Professional Authenticity as a Strategic Advantage

Understanding your masking patterns provides the foundation for strategic authenticity—being more genuinely yourself in professional settings while maintaining career effectiveness. This isn't about abandoning all professional norms but about reducing unnecessary performance that drains your energy without adding value.

Strategic authenticity involves identifying which aspects of professional behavior serve legitimate workplace functions and which exist purely to meet neurotypical social expectations. You can maintain the former while thoughtfully modifying the latter.

Your masking audit reveals specific areas where increased authenticity might actually improve your professional effectiveness. The energy currently spent on performance becomes available for innovation, problem-solving, and genuine relationship building.

Essential Principles for Sustainable Professional Performance

- Professional masking involves sophisticated performance of neurotypical behaviors that consume significant cognitive resources

- Masking-related exhaustion differs from normal work fatigue and requires specific recovery strategies

- Each autistic professional develops unique masking patterns that require individual analysis and intervention

- Strategic authenticity can reduce masking costs while maintaining professional effectiveness

- Systematic tracking provides data needed for optimizing the balance between authenticity and professional requirements

Recognition of masking costs marks the beginning of energy optimization that makes sustainable career success possible. You're ready to explore how reducing masking reveals the professional superpowers that autism provides when your brain operates authentically.

Chapter 3: Autism as a Professional Superpower

The quarterly review meeting was running long, and the team was stuck. Three hours of discussion had produced no clear solution to the production delays that were costing the company $50,000 weekly. Then Sarah, the newly diagnosed autistic quality assurance manager, spoke up from her usual spot at the back of the room. In five minutes, she outlined a systematic analysis that identified the root cause, mapped the interdependencies, and proposed a solution that ultimately saved the company $2.3 million annually.

This wasn't exceptional performance despite her autism—it was exceptional performance because of her autism. Your diagnosis doesn't just explain workplace challenges; it reveals professional advantages that have been hiding in plain sight. The same traits that made certain jobs difficult are the exact qualities that make you exceptionally capable in the right environments.

Systematic Thinking in Complex Business Environments

Your autistic brain approaches problems differently than neurotypical colleagues, and this difference becomes a significant advantage in complex business situations. Where others see overwhelming complexity, you see systems that can be understood, mapped, and optimized.

Pattern recognition allows you to identify connections that others miss. You naturally see how different business functions relate to each other, how changes in one area affect multiple departments, and how small adjustments can produce significant improvements. This systems thinking is exactly what modern organizations need but rarely find.

Consider Mark, a 37-year-old operations analyst who discovered that seemingly unrelated customer complaints all traced back to a single software configuration issue. His autistic brain's tendency to look for underlying patterns revealed that what appeared to be five separate problems was actually one systemic issue. Fixing this root cause improved customer satisfaction scores by 23% and reduced support tickets by 40%.

Logical sequencing helps you understand cause-and-effect relationships that guide effective decision-making. You naturally think through the consequences of business decisions, anticipate potential problems, and develop contingency plans. This systematic approach to planning and problem-solving prevents costly mistakes and ensures thorough implementation.

Process optimization comes naturally to your brain's preference for efficiency and clear structure. You instinctively identify bottlenecks, redundancies, and inefficiencies in business processes. Your suggestions for streamlining operations often produce significant cost savings and productivity improvements.

Jennifer, a 41-year-old project manager, redesigned her company's approval process by mapping every step and identifying unnecessary delays. Her systematic analysis reduced project approval time from six weeks to ten days while improving quality control. The time savings allowed the company to take on 30% more projects without adding staff.

Risk assessment benefits from your tendency to consider multiple variables and potential scenarios. You naturally think about what could go wrong, how likely various problems are, and what mitigation strategies would be most effective. This comprehensive risk analysis helps organizations make informed decisions and avoid costly surprises.

Attention to Detail as a Competitive Advantage

Your natural attention to detail isn't perfectionism or obsessiveness—it's quality control that prevents problems and ensures excellence. In business environments where small errors can have major consequences, your thoroughness becomes an invaluable asset.

Error prevention saves organizations significant money and reputation damage. You catch mistakes before they reach customers, identify compliance issues before they become violations, and spot inconsistencies that could cause problems later. This quality control function is essential but often undervalued until problems occur.

David, a 43-year-old financial analyst, prevented a $3.2 million accounting error by noticing a small discrepancy in quarterly reports that others had missed. His attention to detail didn't just save money—it maintained the company's audit compliance and avoided potential legal issues. His manager later said, "David sees things that the rest of us simply don't notice."

Quality assurance extends beyond catching errors to ensuring that work meets high standards consistently. You maintain quality even under pressure, follow established procedures thoroughly, and produce work that requires minimal revision. This consistency builds trust and reliability that advance your professional reputation.

Documentation excellence reflects your understanding that good records prevent problems and support better decision-making. You create thorough documentation, maintain organized files, and provide clear information that others can use effectively. This documentation often becomes the foundation for improved processes and training materials.

Specification adherence ensures that projects meet their requirements completely. You read instructions carefully, follow procedures systematically, and deliver results that match expectations. This reliability makes you trusted for important projects and complex assignments.

Pattern Recognition for Strategic Planning

Your ability to recognize patterns provides significant advantages in strategic planning and business development. You see trends that others miss, identify opportunities that aren't obvious, and anticipate changes that affect business success.

Market analysis benefits from your systematic approach to data evaluation. You can identify trends in customer behavior, spot opportunities in market research, and recognize patterns in competitive activity. This analysis supports strategic decisions about product development, marketing focus, and business expansion.

Lisa, a 38-year-old marketing manager, analyzed customer service data and identified a pattern showing that customers who used certain product features had 60% higher retention rates. This insight led to changes in onboarding processes and feature promotion that increased overall customer lifetime value by $1.8 million annually.

Predictive planning uses your pattern recognition to anticipate future needs and challenges. You can project how current trends will affect business operations, identify resource requirements before they become critical, and develop strategies for emerging opportunities.

Data interpretation leverages your systematic thinking to extract meaningful insights from complex information sets. You can identify significant patterns in large datasets, recognize anomalies that require attention, and translate data analysis into actionable business recommendations.

Competitive intelligence benefits from your ability to analyze competitor activities systematically and identify patterns in their strategies. You can predict likely competitive responses, identify market gaps, and develop strategies that leverage competitive weaknesses.

Reliability and Consistency as Leadership Qualities

Your natural consistency and systematic approach to work create leadership qualities that organizations desperately need. While others' performance varies based on mood, motivation, or external factors, your systematic approach produces reliable results that build trust and confidence.

Predictable performance allows colleagues and superiors to depend on your work quality and delivery timelines. You meet deadlines consistently, maintain quality standards under pressure, and deliver what you promise. This reliability makes you valuable for critical projects and important client relationships.

Systematic decision-making ensures that your choices are based on logical analysis rather than emotion or impulse. You consider relevant factors thoroughly, evaluate options systematically, and make decisions that can be explained and defended. This approach builds confidence in your judgment and leadership capability.

Robert, a 45-year-old department manager, gained a reputation for making difficult decisions effectively by using a systematic evaluation process. His team knew that his decisions would be fair, well-reasoned, and based on available data rather than personal preferences. This consistency created trust that improved team performance and morale.

Process adherence demonstrates your commitment to organizational standards and continuous improvement. You follow established procedures, maintain quality standards, and suggest improvements based on systematic analysis. This reliability makes you trusted with important responsibilities and complex projects.

Crisis management benefits from your systematic approach to problem-solving and natural tendency to remain calm under pressure. You can analyze crisis situations logically, develop systematic response plans, and implement solutions effectively without being overwhelmed by emotional reactions.

Innovation Through Different Perspectives

Your autism provides a different perspective on business problems that often leads to innovative solutions. Where neurotypical colleagues see standard approaches, you see opportunities for new methods, processes, and strategies.

Creative problem-solving emerges from your tendency to approach problems systematically rather than following conventional wisdom. You're willing to question assumptions, challenge established methods, and explore solutions that others haven't considered. This fresh perspective often produces breakthrough innovations.

Process innovation comes from your natural ability to see how things could work better. You identify inefficiencies in current processes, design improved workflows, and develop systems that increase productivity and quality. Your innovations often seem obvious in retrospect but weren't apparent to others.

Michelle, a 36-year-old software developer, revolutionized her company's testing process by creating automated systems that reduced testing time by 75% while improving error detection. Her systematic approach to the testing problem revealed opportunities for automation that her neurotypical colleagues had missed.

Strategic thinking benefits from your ability to see connections and patterns that inform long-term planning. You can identify how different business factors interact, predict how changes will affect multiple areas, and develop strategies that account for complex interdependencies.

Technology adoption often comes naturally to autistic professionals who appreciate logical systems and efficient processes. You can evaluate new technologies systematically, identify implementation requirements, and develop adoption strategies that maximize benefits while minimizing disruption.

Action Items: Strengths Inventory and Positioning Statement

This systematic assessment helps you identify your specific autistic professional strengths and develop language to communicate these advantages to colleagues and supervisors.

Step 1: Systematic Thinking Assessment Document examples of your systematic thinking in professional settings:

1. **Pattern Recognition Examples**
   - Problems you've solved by identifying underlying patterns
   - Trends you've spotted that others missed
   - Connections you've made between seemingly unrelated issues
   - Predictions you've made that proved accurate

2. **Process Improvement Contributions**
   - Inefficiencies you've identified and addressed
   - Workflows you've streamlined or optimized
   - Quality improvements you've implemented
   - Cost savings resulting from your systematic analysis

3. **Risk Assessment Successes**
   - Problems you've anticipated and prevented

- o Contingency plans you've developed that proved valuable

- o Risk factors you've identified that others overlooked

- o Crisis situations you've managed effectively

Step 2: Detail-Oriented Achievements Catalog specific examples of how your attention to detail created value:

1. **Error Prevention**

   - o Mistakes you've caught before they became problems

   - o Quality issues you've identified and resolved

   - o Compliance problems you've prevented

   - o Financial errors you've discovered and corrected

2. **Quality Assurance**

   - o Projects where your thoroughness ensured success

   - o Standards you've maintained under pressure

   - o Documentation you've created that became valuable resources

   - o Specifications you've followed that prevented problems

Step 3: Innovation Documentation Record instances where your different perspective created innovative solutions:

1. **Creative Solutions**

- Problems you've solved using unconventional approaches
- Processes you've redesigned for better efficiency
- Technologies you've implemented to improve operations
- Strategies you've developed that others hadn't considered

2. **Strategic Contributions**
   - Long-term planning insights you've provided
   - Market opportunities you've identified
   - Competitive advantages you've discovered
   - Business improvements resulting from your analysis

Step 4: Reliability and Consistency Evidence Compile proof of your consistent performance:

1. **Performance Metrics**
   - Deadlines you've met consistently
   - Quality standards you've maintained
   - Productivity measures where you've excelled
   - Client or customer satisfaction related to your work

2. **Leadership Examples**
   - Teams you've led successfully

- Projects you've managed effectively

- Crisis situations you've handled well

- Decisions you've made that produced positive results

Step 5: Professional Positioning Statement Development
Create a clear statement that communicates your autism-based professional strengths:

1. **Core Strengths Summary** Write 2-3 sentences that capture your primary professional advantages:

   - "I bring systematic analytical thinking that identifies root causes and develops comprehensive solutions"

   - "My attention to detail ensures quality and prevents costly errors"

   - "I provide reliable performance and strategic thinking that supports organizational success"

2. **Value Proposition** Develop a statement that connects your strengths to business value:

   - How your systematic thinking saves time and money

   - How your attention to detail prevents problems an

d ensures quality

- How your different perspective drives innovation and improvement
- How your reliability supports project success and team confidence

3. **Professional Brand Integration** Incorporate your strengths into:

   - LinkedIn profile summary
   - Resume objective statements
   - Interview talking points
   - Performance review self-assessments
   - Networking conversations

Step 6: Strength Communication Strategy Develop specific language for different professional contexts:

1. **For Supervisors and Managers**

   - "My systematic approach to problem analysis helps identify root causes that prevent recurring issues"
   - "I consistently deliver high-quality work that meets specifications and deadlines"
   - "My detailed review process catches errors before they reach clients or customers"

2. **For Colleagues and Team Members**

- o "I can help identify patterns in this data that might reveal the underlying issue"

- o "Let me review the specifications to ensure we haven't missed any requirements"

- o "I'd like to suggest a systematic approach to this project that could improve our efficiency"

3. **For Clients and External Partners**

- o "I provide thorough analysis that ensures we understand all aspects of your requirements"

- o "My detailed planning process helps prevent problems and ensures project success"

- o "I bring systematic thinking that identifies opportunities for optimization and improvement"

Leveraging Your Professional Superpowers Strategically

Understanding your autism-based strengths is only the first step—strategic application of these advantages requires intentional positioning and communication. Your goal is to find and create professional situations where your strengths become obvious assets rather than hidden advantages.

Seek high-complexity projects where your systematic thinking provides clear value. Volunteer for assignments that involve process improvement, quality assurance, or strategic analysis. These opportunities allow your autism traits to shine while building your professional reputation.

Position yourself as the detail person on teams and projects. Let colleagues know that you can provide thorough review, catch errors, and ensure quality. This positioning makes your attention to detail a team asset rather than individual perfectionism.

Communicate your analytical approach as a problem-solving methodology rather than personal preference. Frame your systematic thinking as a valuable skill that produces better outcomes, not just how you happen to work.

Build relationships with colleagues who appreciate thoroughness and quality. Seek out mentors and collaborators who value systematic thinking and detailed analysis. These relationships support your professional growth while allowing authentic self-expression.

Transforming Perceived Limitations into Professional Assets

The reframe from autism challenges to autism advantages requires both internal acceptance and external communication. You're not overcoming limitations—you're leveraging natural strengths that happen to operate differently than neurotypical approaches.

Your systematic thinking isn't slow—it's thorough. Your attention to detail isn't perfectionist—it's quality-focused. Your need for clarity isn't rigid—it's precision-oriented. Your direct communication isn't rude—it's efficient. These reframes help you and others understand your autism traits as professional assets.

The key is matching your strengths with appropriate opportunities rather than trying to force them into incompatible situations. A role requiring rapid relationship-building might not suit your social processing style, but a position demanding systematic analysis and quality control perfectly leverages your autism advantages.

Building Your Strength-Based Professional Identity

Your autism diagnosis provides the framework for building a professional identity around authentic strengths rather than masking performance. This shift from hiding differences to leveraging advantages transforms both your career satisfaction and professional effectiveness.

Professional confidence grows when you understand that your brain provides real advantages in business environments. Instead of apologizing for different approaches, you can advocate for methods that produce better results. This confidence attracts opportunities and builds relationships based on mutual value rather than social performance.

Career direction becomes clearer when you understand which environments and roles support your autism strengths. You can make strategic moves toward positions that leverage systematic thinking, attention to detail, and innovation rather than accepting roles that require constant masking.

Leadership development builds on your natural reliability and systematic approach rather than forcing neurotypical leadership styles. You can develop authentic leadership methods that leverage your strengths while acknowledging areas where you might need different strategies or support.

Core Advantages of Autism-Based Professional Success

- Systematic thinking provides advantages in complex business environments that value thorough analysis and strategic planning

- Attention to detail prevents costly errors and ensures quality that builds professional reputation and client trust

- Pattern recognition enables innovation and strategic insights that drive business improvement and competitive advantage

- Reliability and consistency create leadership qualities that organizations desperately need for project success and team stability

- Different perspectives lead to creative solutions and process improvements that neurotypical approaches might miss

Your autism isn't a professional limitation to overcome—it's a set of strengths to leverage strategically. The same traits that made certain jobs difficult are exactly what make you exceptionally capable in the right professional environments.

Understanding these strengths provides the foundation for building authentic professional relationships and creating work environments that support rather than hinder your success. You're ready to assess your specific workplace needs and develop strategies for creating autism-friendly professional environments.

Chapter 4: Understanding Your Workplace Needs

The first day in her new office, Karen noticed everything. The fluorescent lights created a subtle flicker that made reading difficult. The air conditioning system produced a high-pitched whine every twelve minutes. Her desk faced the main walkway, creating constant peripheral movement. The open office design meant conversations from six different workstations competed for her attention simultaneously. By 10:30 AM, she had a headache. By noon, she was exhausted. By 3:00 PM, she was making mistakes on tasks she could normally complete perfectly.

Six months later, after receiving her autism diagnosis, Karen understood what had happened. Her workplace wasn't just uncomfortable—it was neurologically incompatible. Once she understood her specific needs and made targeted modifications, her productivity increased by 40% and her job satisfaction transformed completely.

Sensory Considerations in Office Environments

Your autistic nervous system processes sensory information differently than neurotypical brains, making environmental factors critical determinants of your professional success. What others experience as minor background stimulation can create significant cognitive load that impacts your work performance.

Lighting sensitivity affects many autistic professionals in ways that extend beyond simple discomfort. Fluorescent lights often flicker at frequencies that your brain processes consciously, creating distraction and eye strain. LED lights can produce harsh blue wavelengths that trigger headaches or sensory overload. Natural light variations throughout the day might affect your energy levels and concentration more dramatically than neurotypical colleagues experience.

Michael, a 38-year-old accountant, discovered that his afternoon productivity decline correlated directly with the angle of sunlight hitting his computer screen. The glare created visual stress that progressively degraded his ability to focus on detailed financial data. A simple monitor repositioning and anti-glare screen protector eliminated the problem and maintained his energy levels throughout the day.

Auditory processing challenges in open office environments create multiple layers of cognitive interference. Background conversations, phone calls, keyboard clicking, and HVAC systems all compete for your brain's attention. Unlike neurotypical colleagues who can filter these sounds unconsciously, your brain may process each sound stream separately, creating overwhelming cognitive load.

Temperature and airflow sensitivities can significantly impact your comfort and productivity. You might require more consistent temperatures than others, feel distracted by air movement from vents, or need specific humidity levels for optimal function. These aren't personal preferences— they're neurological requirements for sustained performance.

Tactile considerations include everything from office furniture to clothing requirements. Your desk chair's texture, the keyboard's feel, or carpet textures might create sensory distractions that interfere with work focus. Understanding these tactile needs allows you to make modifications that eliminate unnecessary sensory processing demands.

Olfactory sensitivities can make shared workspaces challenging when colleagues use strong perfumes, eat aromatic foods, or when cleaning products create overwhelming scents. These smells might trigger headaches, nausea, or difficulty concentrating that significantly impacts your work performance.

Communication Preferences and Challenges

Your autism affects how you process and respond to workplace communication, creating both preferences that optimize your performance and challenges that require strategic management. Understanding these patterns allows you to advocate for communication methods that support your success.

Processing time requirements mean you often need more time to formulate responses than typical workplace conversations allow. This isn't slow thinking—it's thorough thinking that considers multiple factors before responding. Quick brainstorming sessions or rapid-fire meetings may not showcase your analytical capabilities effectively.

Sarah, a 35-year-old marketing manager, struggled in weekly team meetings that emphasized quick idea generation and immediate responses. After understanding her processing needs, she requested agenda items in advance and contributed detailed written analysis that informed the team's decisions more effectively than spontaneous verbal input.

Written versus verbal communication preferences often favor written formats that allow processing time and provide permanent reference materials. Email discussions, project documentation, and written proposals may showcase your thinking more effectively than verbal presentations or casual conversations.

Direct communication style reflects your natural tendency toward clarity and efficiency rather than social cushioning. Your straightforward feedback, clear question-asking, and specific information requests can be misinterpreted as rudeness when they're actually attempts at effective communication.

Nonverbal communication differences include variations in eye contact patterns, facial expressions, and body language that don't match neurotypical expectations. These differences don't indicate disinterest or disrespect—they reflect your brain's different social processing patterns.

Meeting participation challenges can arise from multiple factors including sensory overload from conference rooms, difficulty tracking multiple conversation threads, or challenges with the rapid topic changes common in business meetings. Your most valuable contributions might come through different participation formats.

Social Dynamics and Meeting Fatigue

Workplace social interactions require significant energy expenditure for autistic professionals, creating fatigue that impacts both immediate performance and overall job sustainability. Understanding these dynamics helps you manage your energy more effectively.

Small talk energy costs reflect the cognitive load of engaging in conversations that don't serve clear functional purposes. Office chat about weekends, weather, or personal topics requires social script activation and emotional performance that consumes mental resources you could otherwise direct toward work tasks.

Meeting overload occurs when your calendar includes multiple social interactions without adequate recovery time. Back-to-back meetings, especially those requiring high social performance, can create cumulative fatigue that degrades your function throughout the day.

David, a 42-year-old project coordinator, realized that his performance problems on Wednesdays correlated with Tuesday's schedule of five consecutive meetings. The social and sensory demands of extended group interactions created a fatigue that persisted into the following day, affecting his normally excellent analytical work.

Group dynamics navigation requires constant monitoring of social hierarchies, unspoken agendas, and political considerations that can be exhausting to track. Your energy goes toward understanding these dynamics rather than contributing your expertise to the actual business discussion.

Networking event challenges combine sensory overload (noise, crowds, lighting) with intensive social performance requirements. These events can be particularly draining because they require sustained masking without the productivity rewards that make work-related social interaction worthwhile.

Lunch and break expectations for social interaction can eliminate the recovery time you need to sustain performance throughout the day. Your colleagues might interpret your preference for solitary breaks as unfriendliness rather than necessary self-regulation.

Executive Function Support Requirements

Executive function challenges affect how you manage complex tasks, multiple priorities, and time-sensitive deadlines. Understanding these needs allows you to develop support systems that maintain your professional effectiveness.

Task switching difficulties can make environments requiring rapid priority changes particularly challenging. Your brain naturally prefers completing tasks thoroughly before moving to new activities, making interruption-heavy environments less compatible with your optimal performance patterns.

Time management variations might include different estimates for task completion, challenges with scheduling buffer time, or difficulty accurately predicting how long complex projects will require. These aren't planning failures—they're differences in how your brain processes temporal information.

Lisa, a 39-year-old research analyst, discovered that her chronic deadline stress resulted from underestimating the cognitive switching cost between different types of analysis. Once she built transition time into her project schedules, her work quality improved and her stress levels decreased significantly.

Organization system requirements often differ from standard workplace approaches. You might need more detailed filing systems, specific project tracking methods, or particular environmental organization to maintain optimal function. These systems aren't excessive—they're necessary supports for your cognitive processing style.

Priority management challenges can arise when workplace demands compete for your attention without clear hierarchy or importance ranking. Your systematic thinking works best with clear priorities and logical task sequences rather than ambiguous or constantly changing demands.

Deadline pressure responses might differ from neurotypical patterns, with some autistic professionals performing better with extended timelines while others work more effectively with structured deadline pressure. Understanding your optimal pressure levels allows you to negotiate appropriate project timelines.

Action Items: Workplace Needs Assessment

This systematic evaluation helps you identify specific environmental, communication, and support needs that optimize your professional performance.

Environmental Assessment Protocol

1. **Sensory Environment Audit** For one week, track how environmental factors affect your energy and performance:

Lighting Impact Tracking

- Rate your energy level hourly on days with different lighting conditions
- Note headaches, eye strain, or concentration difficulties related to lighting
- Identify optimal lighting conditions for different types of work

- Document times when lighting changes affect your performance

Sound Environment Analysis

- Record background noise levels and types throughout your workday

- Note correlation between noise levels and concentration ability

- Identify sounds that are particularly distracting or energizing

- Track how sound changes affect your work quality and speed

Physical Comfort Evaluation

- Monitor temperature, airflow, and seating comfort throughout the day

- Note physical discomfort that affects concentration

- Identify optimal physical conditions for sustained focus

- Document ergonomic factors that impact your performance

2. **Communication Pattern Analysis** For one week, analyze your communication effectiveness:

Processing Time Documentation

- Note meetings or conversations where you needed more processing time

- Track situations where quick responses were required vs. preferred
- Identify communication formats that showcase your thinking most effectively
- Record instances where processing time affected your contribution quality

Communication Format Preferences

- Compare your effectiveness in written vs. verbal communication
- Note which communication styles feel most natural and productive
- Track energy costs of different communication types
- Identify communication situations that require significant masking

Social and Executive Function Assessment

3. **Social Energy Tracking** Monitor the energy costs of workplace social interactions:

Meeting Impact Analysis

- Rate your energy before and after different types of meetings
- Track how meeting frequency affects your daily performance
- Note which meeting formats are most and least draining

o   Identify optimal spacing between social interactions

Social Performance Costs

o   Document energy required for small talk and casual interactions

o   Track how networking events or social expectations affect your recovery time

o   Note correlation between social demands and work performance

o   Identify social interactions that feel natural vs. performative

4. **Executive Function Evaluation** Assess how workplace demands align with your cognitive processing:

Task Management Analysis

o   Track your effectiveness with different task switching frequencies

o   Note optimal task duration and complexity for sustained focus

o   Identify organizational systems that support vs. hinder your productivity

o   Document how interruptions affect your work quality and completion time

Priority and Deadline Assessment

o   Analyze how you respond to different deadline structures

- Track your accuracy in estimating task completion times
- Note how competing priorities affect your decision-making and stress levels
- Identify optimal workload distribution throughout your day and week

Needs Summary and Prioritization

5. **Critical Needs Identification** Based on your assessment data, identify:

High-Impact Environmental Modifications

- Sensory changes that would significantly improve your performance
- Communication adjustments that would reduce energy costs
- Social interaction modifications that would support sustainability

Moderate-Impact Improvements

- Changes that would improve comfort and efficiency
- Adjustments that would reduce daily stress and fatigue
- Modifications that would enhance job satisfaction

Nice-to-Have Preferences

- Changes that would optimize your performance beyond basic needs

- Environmental improvements that would maximize your professional strengths
- Support systems that would enable exceptional performance

6. **Implementation Strategy Development** Create specific plans for addressing your identified needs:

Immediate Self-Modifications

- Changes you can make independently without requiring approval
- Environmental adjustments within your control
- Communication strategies you can implement immediately

Supervisor Discussion Items

- Needs that require manager approval or support
- Modifications that might require modest resource investment
- Changes that could be framed as productivity improvements

Formal Accommodation Requests

- Significant environmental or role modifications
- Changes that require HR involvement or formal documentation

○ Accommodations that might require policy adjustments

Creating Your Optimal Work Environment

Understanding your workplace needs provides the foundation for creating professional environments that support rather than hinder your autism strengths. This isn't about demanding special treatment—it's about optimizing conditions for maximum productivity and job satisfaction.

Environmental optimization focuses on modifications that reduce sensory processing demands and create conditions where your concentration and analytical abilities can flourish. These changes often benefit neurotypical colleagues as well, making them easier to implement and sustain.

Communication strategy development involves advocating for interaction styles that showcase your strengths while managing your processing needs. This might include requesting meeting agendas in advance, contributing written analysis alongside verbal discussion, or scheduling focused work time between social interactions.

Energy management planning helps you structure your workday and week to account for the varying energy costs of different activities. This strategic approach to energy allocation ensures that you can sustain high performance while avoiding the burnout that comes from unmanaged social and sensory demands.

Essential Elements for Autism-Friendly Professional Environments

- Environmental modifications that reduce sensory processing load significantly improve concentration and energy management

- Communication strategies that accommodate processing time and style preferences showcase autism strengths more effectively

- Social interaction management prevents the fatigue that degrades performance and threatens job sustainability

- Executive function supports enable complex task management while working with rather than against autism cognitive patterns

- Systematic assessment of specific needs provides data for targeted modifications that optimize professional performance

Your workplace needs aren't personal preferences or special requirements—they're professional optimization strategies that enable your autism strengths to contribute effectively to organizational success. Understanding these needs prepares you for the strategic decisions about disclosure and accommodation that can transform your career experience.

Path Forward to Professional Success

Recognition of your specific workplace needs marks a turning point in your professional journey. You're no longer trying to adapt yourself to incompatible environments— you're developing strategies to create conditions where your autism strengths can flourish.

This assessment provides the foundation for every subsequent decision about accommodation requests, job changes, and career planning. You now have data about what works, what doesn't, and why. This knowledge becomes your guide for building a sustainable and satisfying professional life that honors your neurological differences while achieving your career goals.

Your next step involves translating this self-awareness into strategic action through disclosure decisions, accommodation requests, and workplace modifications that create the environment where your professional superpowers can transform both your success and your organization's outcomes.

Key Insights for Professional Development

- Sensory environment optimization significantly impacts concentration, energy, and performance quality

- Communication preferences reflect processing differences that can be leveraged as professional strengths

- Social interaction management prevents energy depletion that compromises work effectiveness

- Executive function support systems enable complex task management while honoring autism cognitive patterns

- Systematic needs assessment provides concrete data for implementing workplace modifications that benefit both individual and organizational success

Chapter 5: The Strategic Disclosure Decision

The email sat in Jennifer's drafts folder for three weeks. "Subject: Accommodation Request - Autism Diagnosis." She'd written and rewritten it seventeen times, each version attempting to strike the perfect balance between professional necessity and personal vulnerability. As a senior analyst at a Fortune 500 company, she understood risk assessment better than most. But this decision felt different—more personal, more consequential, and more uncertain than any business choice she'd ever made.

Jennifer's hesitation wasn't unusual. The disclosure decision represents one of the most complex calculations that late-diagnosed autistic professionals face. You're weighing legal protections against potential discrimination, professional benefits against personal exposure, and immediate needs against long-term career implications. This decision requires strategic thinking, not emotional impulses.

The Disclosure Decision Tree - Factors to Consider

Effective disclosure decisions require systematic analysis of multiple variables that interact in complex ways. Your choice isn't simply about comfort level or personal preference—it's a strategic calculation that affects your career trajectory, daily work experience, and professional relationships.

Current job security forms the foundation of your disclosure analysis. Employees with strong performance records, specialized skills, or significant tenure have different risk profiles than those in probationary periods or performance improvement plans. Your individual value to the organization affects how your disclosure will be received and what accommodations are likely to be approved.

Consider Michael, a 41-year-old software architect with eight years at his company and expertise in legacy systems that only three people in the organization understood. His specialized knowledge and proven track record provided significant protection when he disclosed his autism diagnosis and requested environmental accommodations. The company viewed his needs as minor adjustments to retain essential expertise.

Industry culture and organizational attitudes toward diversity and inclusion vary dramatically across sectors and individual companies. Progressive technology companies often embrace neurodiversity as innovation drivers, while traditional industries might view autism disclosure with more skepticism. Research your organization's actual track record with accommodations, not just their published policies.

Accommodation necessity helps determine disclosure urgency. If your current workplace challenges are manageable through personal strategies, you might delay disclosure until your situation changes. However, if sensory overload, communication difficulties, or executive function challenges significantly impact your performance, earlier disclosure becomes strategically necessary.

Career stage considerations affect how disclosure fits into your professional trajectory. Early-career professionals might benefit from establishing accommodation patterns that support long-term success, while senior professionals might focus on disclosure timing that doesn't interfere with advancement opportunities or leadership responsibilities.

Sarah, a 38-year-old marketing director, delayed disclosure until after receiving a promotion she'd worked toward for two years. The timing allowed her to establish credibility in her new role before requesting accommodations that supported her continued success. Her strategic delay paid off when her supervisor viewed her accommodation needs as productivity optimization rather than performance deficits.

Team dynamics and manager relationships significantly influence disclosure outcomes. Supportive managers who value your contributions will likely view accommodation requests favorably, while managers focused on compliance over performance might create more challenging implementation experiences.

Legal and documentation status of your autism diagnosis affects the formal protections available to you. Official diagnoses from licensed professionals provide stronger legal foundations for accommodation requests than self-diagnosis or informal assessments, even though all autism experiences are valid.

Legal Protections and Potential Risks

Understanding your legal rights and protections under disability law provides the framework for making informed disclosure decisions. These protections are substantial but not absolute, and knowing both their scope and limitations helps you assess your disclosure risk accurately.

Americans with Disabilities Act (ADA) coverage extends to autism spectrum conditions when they substantially limit major life activities. The law requires employers to provide reasonable accommodations unless they create undue hardship for the organization (1). This protection applies to companies with fifteen or more employees and covers most professional work environments.

Reasonable accommodation requirements obligate employers to modify work environments, schedules, or responsibilities to enable qualified employees to perform essential job functions. Examples include sensory modifications, schedule adjustments, communication preferences, and task restructuring. The key legal standard is "reasonable"—accommodations that don't fundamentally alter job requirements or impose excessive costs.

David, a 43-year-old financial analyst, successfully requested noise-canceling headphones, a private office space, and written rather than verbal project instructions. These accommodations cost his employer less than $500 but improved his productivity by 35%. The clear business benefit made the accommodations easily defensible under ADA requirements.

Anti-retaliation protections prohibit employers from taking adverse actions against employees who request accommodations or file discrimination complaints. This includes protection against termination, demotion, harassment, or other negative treatment related to your disclosure or accommodation needs.

Documentation requirements for ADA protection typically include professional diagnosis and medical documentation of your condition's impact on work-related activities. Your accommodation requests must connect specifically to autism-related challenges that affect job performance or workplace experience.

Potential risks and limitations exist despite legal protections. Discrimination can be subtle and difficult to prove. Some managers might become uncomfortable with your differences even while formally complying with accommodation requirements. Career advancement opportunities might be affected by colleagues' or supervisors' unconscious biases about autism capabilities.

State and local protections often provide additional safeguards beyond federal ADA requirements. Many states have stronger disability rights laws, lower employee thresholds for coverage, or enhanced anti-discrimination protections. Research your specific jurisdiction's laws for complete protection understanding.

Timing Your Disclosure for Maximum Benefit

Strategic disclosure timing maximizes the benefits of legal protections while minimizing potential negative consequences. The optimal timing depends on your specific circumstances, but certain principles guide effective disclosure strategies.

Post-hire timing generally provides stronger protection than pre-hire disclosure. Once you've demonstrated job competence and received positive performance feedback, your autism diagnosis becomes context for optimizing already-proven capabilities rather than potential limitations on unknown abilities.

Performance review cycles offer natural opportunities for disclosure conversations. Strong performance evaluations provide evidence of your capabilities while creating openings to discuss how accommodations could further improve your contributions. This timing frames accommodation requests as productivity enhancements rather than problem solutions.

Lisa, a 36-year-old project manager, timed her disclosure to coincide with her annual review meeting where she received exceptional ratings in all categories. She presented her autism diagnosis as additional context for understanding her systematic approach to project management and requested specific accommodations that would allow her to take on more complex assignments.

Before accommodation needs become critical allows proactive planning rather than crisis management. If you can anticipate upcoming challenges—new office moves, team restructuring, increased travel requirements—early disclosure enables collaborative solution development rather than emergency accommodation requests.

During positive relationship periods with supervisors creates better foundation for accommodation discussions. If you have strong working relationships and recent professional successes, disclosure conversations occur in positive rather than defensive contexts.

Project completion timing avoids disclosure during high-stress periods when managers are focused on immediate deliverables rather than long-term employee development. Choose periods when your supervisor has mental space for thoughtful accommodation discussions.

Avoid timing during organizational stress periods, budget constraints, layoffs, or management transitions. These circumstances increase resistance to accommodation requests and reduce the mental resources available for supportive responses to your disclosure.

Who Needs to Know and Who Doesn't

Strategic disclosure involves sharing information with people who need to know while maintaining privacy with those who don't. This selective approach protects your personal information while ensuring that relevant parties can provide necessary support.

Direct supervisor requirements typically include disclosure for accommodation implementation and performance management purposes. Your immediate manager needs enough information to understand your needs and approve necessary workplace modifications, but they don't require detailed medical information about your diagnosis.

Human Resources notification is usually necessary for formal accommodation processes and legal documentation. HR professionals handle disability accommodation procedures and ensure compliance with organizational policies and legal requirements. They maintain confidentiality while coordinating accommodation implementation.

Accommodation implementers need specific information about your needs without requiring full disclosure of your autism diagnosis. Facilities managers arranging workspace modifications, IT staff providing assistive technology, or schedulers adjusting meeting formats need functional information rather than diagnostic details.

Mark, a 39-year-old operations manager, informed his supervisor about his autism diagnosis and need for specific accommodations, provided HR with required medical documentation, and gave facilities management specific environmental requirements without mentioning autism. This selective disclosure achieved his accommodation goals while limiting unnecessary personal exposure.

Team members generally don't need autism disclosure unless your accommodations directly affect their work or you choose personal sharing for relationship-building purposes. Many accommodations (noise-canceling headphones, schedule modifications, communication preferences) don't require team explanation or disclosure.

Clients and external partners rarely need autism disclosure unless your accommodations affect external meetings or communication patterns. Professional accommodation needs can usually be addressed through standard business communication about preferences and requirements.

Professional network contacts don't require disclosure unless you choose to advocate for autism awareness or build relationships with other neurodivergent professionals. Disclosure to mentors, career coaches, or professional organizations is personal choice rather than strategic necessity.

Scripts for Different Disclosure Scenarios

Effective disclosure conversations require preparation and clear language that focuses on accommodation needs rather than diagnostic details. These scripts provide frameworks that you can adapt to your specific situation and communication style.

Initial Disclosure to Direct Supervisor

"I wanted to discuss some workplace accommodations that would help me maintain my performance level and take on additional responsibilities. I've recently been diagnosed with autism, which explains some of the work patterns you've probably noticed. I'm requesting a few specific modifications that will allow me to continue contributing effectively to our team goals."

This script establishes the business focus, connects to known performance patterns, and frames accommodations as productivity enhancements rather than problem solutions.

Formal HR Accommodation Request

"I'm submitting a formal accommodation request under the Americans with Disabilities Act. I have been diagnosed with Autism Spectrum Disorder, which affects my sensory processing and communication preferences. I'm requesting the following specific accommodations that will enable me to perform my essential job functions effectively: [specific list]. I have medical documentation available to support this request."

This script uses proper legal language, focuses on essential job functions, and provides clear accommodation specifications for HR processing.

Follow-up Discussion with Supervisor

"I wanted to check in about how the accommodations are working and whether you've noticed any impact on my productivity or team contributions. I'm happy to adjust the arrangements if needed to ensure they're meeting both my needs and our department goals."

This script demonstrates ongoing collaboration and commitment to team success while maintaining accommodation effectiveness.

Accommodation Modification Request

"I'd like to discuss modifying one of my current accommodations based on how it's working in practice. The [specific accommodation] has been helpful, but I think [specific modification] would be even more effective for [specific business outcome]. Can we explore this adjustment?"

This script shows accommodation flexibility and continued focus on business results rather than personal preferences.

Team Communication (if needed)

"I wanted to let you know that I'll be using [specific accommodation] going forward. This change will help me maintain my focus and productivity while contributing to our team projects. It shouldn't affect our collaboration, but please let me know if you have any questions about how we can work together effectively."

This script provides necessary information without detailed disclosure while maintaining professional relationships and team cooperation.

Action Items: Disclosure Readiness Checklist

This systematic assessment helps you determine your readiness for disclosure and develop an effective disclosure strategy based on your specific circumstances.

Situation Assessment Phase

1. **Job Security Evaluation**

- o Rate your current job security on a 1-10 scale based on performance reviews, tenure, and specialized skills

- o Document recent performance feedback and achievement recognition

- o Assess your value to the organization based on expertise and contribution uniqueness

- o Identify any current performance concerns or improvement plans

2. **Organizational Culture Analysis**

- o Research your company's diversity and inclusion policies and actual implementation

- o Identify other employees who have received accommodations and their experiences

- o Assess your manager's leadership style and openness to employee needs

- o Evaluate HR department's reputation for handling sensitive employee issues

3. **Accommodation Necessity Assessment**

- o List specific workplace challenges that accommodations would address

- o Rate the urgency of each accommodation need on a 1-5 scale

- o Document how current challenges affect your work performance

- Identify temporary solutions you're currently using and their sustainability

Legal and Documentation Preparation

4. **Documentation Review**

   - Confirm you have official autism diagnosis from licensed professional

   - Gather medical records that document work-related functional impacts

   - Review your company's accommodation policies and procedures

   - Identify specific ADA protections relevant to your situation

5. **Accommodation Planning**

   - List specific accommodations you need with clear business justifications

   - Research cost and implementation requirements for each accommodation

   - Develop alternative accommodation options for flexibility in negotiations

   - Connect each accommodation to specific job functions and performance improvements

Strategic Timing Analysis

6. **Timing Optimization**

   - Identify optimal disclosure timing based on performance cycles and relationship status

- Avoid periods of organizational stress, budget constraints, or management transitions
- Plan disclosure around positive performance feedback or project completions
- Schedule adequate time for accommodation implementation and adjustment

7. **Communication Planning**

- Decide who needs full disclosure versus functional information only
- Prepare disclosure scripts adapted to your communication style
- Plan follow-up conversations and accommodation effectiveness discussions
- Develop strategies for handling potential negative responses or questions

Risk Mitigation Preparation

8. **Backup Planning**

- Identify alternative career options if disclosure creates workplace problems
- Research other autism-friendly employers in your field
- Update professional credentials and portfolio documentation
- Build professional network connections for potential job search support

9. **Support System Development**

- Identify colleagues, mentors, or advocates who can provide professional support

- Connect with autism support organizations or professional networks

- Research legal resources for discrimination issues if needed

- Plan personal support strategies for managing disclosure stress

Implementation Strategy Finalization

10. **Disclosure Decision Matrix** Based on your assessment, rate each factor:

     - Job security strength (1-5)

     - Organizational culture supportiveness (1-5)

     - Accommodation urgency (1-5)

     - Legal protection confidence (1-5)

     - Timing optimization (1-5)

Total scores above 20 suggest disclosure readiness, while scores below 15 indicate need for additional preparation or situational improvement.

Moving Forward with Confidence

Your disclosure decision affects not just your immediate work experience but your long-term career trajectory and professional satisfaction. This strategic approach ensures that your choice is based on careful analysis rather than emotional impulses or external pressure.

The goal isn't to find the "right" decision that works for everyone—it's to find the right decision for your specific situation, career goals, and personal values. Some professionals thrive with full disclosure and accommodation implementation, while others succeed with minimal disclosure and self-managed strategies.

Your disclosure timing and approach can always be adjusted as circumstances change. Initial decisions aren't permanent commitments, and you can modify your strategy as you gain experience, change roles, or encounter new situations.

Strategic Implementation Success

- Effective disclosure decisions require systematic analysis of job security, organizational culture, accommodation necessity, and legal protections

- Timing disclosure strategically maximizes benefits while minimizing potential negative consequences

- Selective disclosure shares information with people who need to know while protecting privacy with others

- Prepared scripts and clear accommodation requests increase success rates and professional credibility

- Systematic readiness assessment ensures decisions are based on facts rather than emotions

Your disclosure decision represents a turning point in your professional journey from hiding differences to leveraging strengths. You're ready to translate this strategic foundation into specific accommodation requests that create work environments where your autism becomes a professional advantage

Chapter 6: Requesting Accommodations That Work

The accommodation request form stared back at Rachel from her computer screen, cursor blinking in the empty "Requested Accommodations" field. Three weeks had passed since her autism diagnosis, and the fluorescent lights in her cubicle continued triggering daily headaches. Her manager's rapid-fire meeting style left her confused and overwhelmed. The open office chaos made concentration nearly impossible. She knew what she needed—she just didn't know how to ask for it professionally.

Six months later, Rachel worked in a quiet corner office with natural lighting, received meeting agendas in advance, and had become her department's most productive analyst. The transformation didn't happen by accident. It resulted from strategic accommodation requests that connected her autism needs to business benefits while following proven implementation processes.

Understanding Your Rights Under the ADA

The Americans with Disabilities Act provides specific protections for qualified employees with disabilities, including autism spectrum conditions. Understanding these rights forms the foundation for effective accommodation requests that protect your interests while meeting legal requirements (1).

Qualified individual status requires that you can perform the essential functions of your job with or without reasonable accommodations. Your autism diagnosis alone doesn't determine qualification—your ability to fulfill core job responsibilities does. This distinction is significant because it focuses accommodation discussions on job performance rather than diagnostic categories.

Essential function determination involves identifying which job duties are fundamental and which are peripheral. Essential functions are usually listed in job descriptions, represent major portions of work time, or require specialized skills that justify the position's existence. Accommodations cannot eliminate essential functions but can modify how you perform them.

Consider Tom, a 42-year-old accountant whose essential functions included financial analysis, report preparation, and regulatory compliance. His accommodation request for quiet workspace and written communication preferences didn't change these core responsibilities but modified how he accomplished them more effectively.

Reasonable accommodation scope covers modifications or adjustments that enable you to perform essential job functions without creating undue hardship for your employer. The law defines reasonable accommodations broadly to include environmental changes, schedule modifications, equipment provision, and policy adjustments (1).

Interactive process requirements obligate both you and your employer to engage in collaborative problem-solving to identify effective accommodations. This isn't a one-sided demand process—it's a cooperative effort to find solutions that meet your needs while serving business interests.

Undue hardship limitations allow employers to deny accommodation requests that create significant difficulty or expense relative to their size and resources. However, this standard is high—most autism-related accommodations involve minimal cost and create measurable productivity benefits.

Confidentiality protections require employers to keep your medical information separate from personnel files and limit access to people who need accommodation implementation information. Your supervisor might know you need specific environmental modifications without knowing your autism diagnosis details.

Identifying Effective Accommodations for Your Role

Successful accommodation requests connect your specific autism needs to concrete workplace modifications that improve your performance while addressing business objectives. Generic accommodation lists rarely work— effective requests reflect your individual challenges and job requirements.

Sensory environment modifications address the environmental factors that affect your concentration and energy levels. These accommodations often provide immediate relief while supporting long-term productivity improvements.

- **Lighting adjustments** including desk lamps to reduce fluorescent exposure, window positioning to control glare, or office relocation to areas with natural light

- **Sound management** through noise-canceling headphones, white noise machines, or workspace relocation away from high-traffic areas

- **Temperature and airflow control** via personal fans, heating devices, or seating arrangements that avoid direct HVAC exposure

- **Workspace organization** including private offices, cubicle modifications, or designated quiet work areas

Communication accommodations optimize how you receive and process work-related information while maintaining collaborative effectiveness.

- **Written communication preferences** for meeting follow-ups, project instructions, and feedback delivery

- **Advance notice for meetings** including agendas, objectives, and preparation materials

- **Processing time allowances** for complex decisions or detailed responses

- **Alternative meeting formats** such as one-on-one discussions instead of large group sessions

Sarah, a 37-year-old project manager, requested written project specifications and 24-hour notice for urgent meetings. These accommodations improved her project delivery time by 30% because she could process information thoroughly before responding.

Schedule and routine accommodations support your executive function needs while maintaining productivity and collaboration requirements.

- **Flexible work hours** to accommodate your optimal performance periods

- **Break scheduling** that allows sensory recovery and energy management

- **Deadline structure** with clear milestones and buffer time for complex projects

- **Task organization** support through project management tools or administrative assistance

Technology accommodations leverage assistive tools that improve your work efficiency and reduce cognitive load.

- **Organizational software** for task management, calendar coordination, and project tracking

- **Communication tools** that support your preferred interaction styles

- **Environmental controls** like adjustable lighting or sound management devices

- **Accessibility features** in standard software applications

How to Present Accommodation Requests Professionally

Professional accommodation requests frame your autism needs as productivity optimization opportunities rather than problem-solving requirements. This approach increases approval likelihood while establishing collaborative relationships with supervisors and HR staff.

Business benefits focus connects each accommodation to specific performance improvements or organizational advantages. Your request should demonstrate how modifications will improve your contributions to team and company goals.

Documentation structure for accommodation requests should include clear identification of needs, specific modification requests, implementation suggestions, and success metrics. This systematic approach helps HR and management understand both your requirements and their obligations.

Professional language guidelines avoid medical jargon or emotional appeals in favor of clear, business-focused communication. Your request should sound like a process improvement proposal rather than a personal plea for special treatment.

Here's an effective accommodation request framework:

"I am requesting workplace accommodations under the Americans with Disabilities Act to optimize my performance in my role as [position title]. I have been diagnosed with Autism Spectrum Disorder, which affects my sensory processing and communication style. The following accommodations will enable me to perform my essential job functions more effectively:

1. **Quiet workspace or noise-reducing equipment** to minimize sensory distractions that impact concentration on detailed analysis tasks

2. **Written meeting summaries and advance agendas** to ensure I can prepare effectively and contribute meaningfully to team discussions

3. **Flexible scheduling for deep focus work** during my most productive hours to maximize output quality

These modifications support my proven strengths in [specific skills] while addressing environmental factors that can impact my performance. I believe these accommodations will result in [specific business benefits]. I have medical documentation available to support this request and am happy to discuss implementation details."

Cost-effectiveness emphasis demonstrates that your accommodations provide positive return on investment through improved productivity, quality, or efficiency. Many autism accommodations cost less than $500 while producing significant performance improvements (2).

Implementation suggestions show that you've thought through practical aspects of accommodation delivery. Offering specific solutions demonstrates professionalism while making approval easier for decision-makers.

Flexibility demonstration indicates your willingness to collaborate on accommodation details and adjust approaches based on business needs. This cooperative attitude encourages positive responses and ongoing support.

Working with HR to Implement Changes

Human Resources departments handle accommodation requests through structured processes designed to ensure legal compliance while meeting business needs. Understanding these processes helps you navigate implementation more effectively while building supportive relationships.

Initial documentation requirements typically include formal request submission, medical verification of your diagnosis, and functional impact statements that connect your autism to work-related challenges. Prepare these materials carefully because they form the legal foundation for your accommodations.

Interactive process participation involves collaborative discussions about accommodation options, implementation timelines, and effectiveness measures. HR professionals are required to engage in good faith problem-solving rather than simply approving or denying requests.

David, a 44-year-old marketing analyst, worked with HR to modify his initial accommodation request when the first proposal proved impractical. Instead of a private office (which wasn't available), they arranged a quiet workspace with environmental controls and flexible scheduling that achieved the same concentration benefits.

Implementation coordination requires HR to work with facilities, IT, management, and other departments to deliver approved accommodations. Your role involves providing feedback about effectiveness and suggesting adjustments as needed.

Documentation maintenance includes keeping records of accommodation discussions, implementation steps, and effectiveness assessments. This documentation protects both you and your employer while supporting future accommodation modifications.

Effectiveness monitoring involves regular check-ins with HR and your supervisor to assess how accommodations are working and identify needed adjustments. This ongoing process ensures that modifications continue meeting your needs as job requirements or circumstances change.

Confidentiality management means HR limits access to your medical information while coordinating accommodation implementation. Your supervisor might know you need specific modifications without knowing diagnostic details.

Documenting Your Accommodation Needs

Thorough documentation creates the foundation for successful accommodation requests while protecting your rights throughout the implementation process. This documentation serves legal, practical, and communication purposes that support long-term success.

Medical documentation requirements include official diagnosis from licensed professionals, functional impact assessments that connect autism to work challenges, and treatment provider recommendations for specific accommodations. This documentation establishes your legal right to accommodations under ADA requirements.

Work impact documentation demonstrates how autism affects your job performance and workplace experience. This might include examples of sensory overload affecting concentration, communication challenges impacting meeting participation, or executive function difficulties with task management.

Lisa, a 35-year-old operations coordinator, documented specific instances where open office noise reduced her data entry accuracy by 25% and increased error rates. This concrete evidence supported her request for quiet workspace accommodations and demonstrated clear business benefits.

Accommodation effectiveness tracking monitors how modifications affect your performance, energy levels, and job satisfaction. This ongoing documentation supports accommodation adjustments and provides evidence for future requests or role changes.

Communication records include correspondence with HR, supervisor discussions about accommodations, and implementation feedback. These records protect your interests while demonstrating collaborative engagement with accommodation processes.

Performance correlation analysis connects accommodation implementation to measurable improvements in work quality, productivity, or efficiency. This data supports the business case for continued accommodation provision and potential expansion.

Action Items: Accommodation Request Template and Tracker

This systematic approach helps you develop professional accommodation requests and track their implementation effectiveness over time.

Pre-Request Preparation Phase

1. **Needs Assessment Documentation** Create detailed records of your specific accommodation needs:

Sensory Environment Challenges

- List specific environmental factors that affect your performance
- Document times when sensory issues impact work quality or efficiency
- Rate severity of different environmental challenges on 1-5 scale

- Identify patterns in sensory overload and recovery requirements

Communication and Social Accommodation Needs

- Document communication preferences that optimize your performance
- Record instances where communication style differences affect work outcomes
- List social interaction accommodations that would reduce energy costs
- Identify meeting formats that best support your participation

Executive Function Support Requirements

- List organizational and planning challenges that affect work performance
- Document time management difficulties and their impact on deadlines
- Identify task management supports that would improve efficiency
- Record attention and focus challenges that accommodations could address

2. **Job Function Analysis** Map your accommodation needs to essential job functions:

Essential Function Identification

- List all essential job duties from your position description

- Identify which functions are affected by autism-related challenges
- Document how accommodations would improve essential function performance
- Distinguish essential functions from peripheral job duties

Performance Impact Assessment

- Rate how autism challenges affect each essential job function
- Document specific examples of performance impact
- Identify accommodation solutions for each affected function
- Calculate potential performance improvements from accommodations

Formal Request Development

3. **Accommodation Request Template** Use this structure for professional accommodation requests:

Header Information

- Your name, position title, and department
- Date of request submission
- Supervisor and HR contact information
- Reference to Americans with Disabilities Act

Diagnosis Disclosure Statement "I am requesting workplace accommodations under the Americans with

Disabilities Act. I have been diagnosed with Autism Spectrum Disorder by [licensed professional type]. This condition affects [specific functional areas] in ways that impact my work performance."

Specific Accommodation Requests For each accommodation, include:

- Clear description of requested modification
- Connection to specific job function or workplace challenge
- Business benefit or performance improvement expected
- Implementation suggestions or alternatives
- Estimated cost or resource requirements (if known)

Business Benefits Summary "These accommodations will enable me to [specific performance improvements] while contributing to [team/department/company goals]. Based on my current performance patterns, I expect these modifications will result in [measurable benefits]."

Implementation Collaboration "I am committed to working collaboratively with HR and my supervisor to implement these accommodations effectively. I'm happy to provide additional information, adjust approaches based on business needs, and participate in regular effectiveness reviews."

4. **Supporting Documentation Package** Compile materials that support your request:

Medical Documentation

- Official diagnosis letter from licensed professional
- Functional impact assessment connecting autism to work challenges
- Treatment provider recommendations for specific accommodations
- Any additional medical records that support accommodation needs

Work Performance Evidence

- Performance reviews showing your job competence
- Examples of work quality or achievements
- Documentation of current challenges and their impact
- Evidence of how similar accommodations have helped in past situations

Implementation Tracking System

5. **Accommodation Implementation Tracker** Monitor progress through systematic tracking:

Request Status Tracking

- Date of initial request submission
- HR acknowledgment and timeline estimates
- Interactive process meeting dates and outcomes

- Approval notifications and implementation schedules
- Any delays or complications and their resolutions

Implementation Progress Monitoring

- Specific accommodations approved vs. requested
- Implementation start dates for each accommodation
- Completion status and any ongoing adjustments needed
- Resource allocation and actual costs (if available)
- Timeline adherence and communication effectiveness

6. **Effectiveness Assessment Protocol** Evaluate accommodation success systematically:

Performance Impact Measurement

- Baseline performance metrics before accommodation implementation
- Performance measures after accommodation implementation
- Specific improvements in work quality, speed, or efficiency
- Energy level changes and sustainability improvements

- Any unexpected benefits or challenges from accommodations

Adjustment and Optimization Tracking

- Accommodation modifications needed after initial implementation

- Seasonal or situation-specific adjustment requirements

- Communication effectiveness with supervisors and HR

- Ongoing collaboration success and relationship impacts

- Long-term accommodation sustainability and success patterns

Ongoing Management Strategy

7. **Accommodation Review and Update Process**
   Maintain accommodation effectiveness over time:

Regular Review Schedule

- Monthly self-assessment of accommodation effectiveness

- Quarterly supervisor discussions about accommodation impacts

- Annual formal review with HR for documentation updates

- Job change or role modification accommodation assessments

Continuous Improvement Framework

- Feedback collection from supervisors and colleagues

- Identification of accommodation gaps or additional needs

- Success story documentation for future requests

- Professional development planning that incorporates accommodation needs

Building Long-Term Accommodation Success

Effective accommodation implementation extends beyond initial approval to ongoing management that ensures continued effectiveness as your role and circumstances change. This long-term perspective helps you build sustainable professional success while maintaining positive relationships with supervisors and colleagues.

Accommodation evolution acknowledges that your needs might change as you gain experience, take on new responsibilities, or encounter different workplace challenges. Regular effectiveness reviews ensure that modifications continue supporting your optimal performance.

Professional relationship maintenance involves demonstrating how accommodations improve your contributions while maintaining collaborative relationships with colleagues and supervisors. Your accommodations should enhance rather than complicate team dynamics and work processes.

Career advancement planning considers how accommodations transfer to new roles or responsibilities and how disclosure affects promotion opportunities. Strategic planning ensures that accommodation needs don't inadvertently limit your career growth or professional development.

Pathway to Professional Optimization

- ADA protections provide substantial rights to reasonable accommodations that enable you to perform essential job functions effectively

- Successful accommodation requests connect autism needs to specific business benefits while following professional documentation standards

- HR collaboration requires systematic preparation and ongoing communication that demonstrates cooperative problem-solving

- Thorough documentation protects your rights while supporting accommodation effectiveness and future modifications

- Strategic implementation creates work environments where autism becomes a professional advantage rather than a challenge

Your accommodation success transforms not just your immediate work experience but your long-term career trajectory and professional satisfaction. You're ready to address specific sensory challenges that often form the foundation of autism workplace difficulties.

Chapter 7: Managing Sensory Challenges in Professional Settings

The quarterly board presentation was scheduled for 2:00 PM in the executive conference room—the one with floor-to-ceiling windows facing west, chrome fixtures that reflected fluorescent lights, and a ventilation system that hummed at precisely the frequency that made Alex's skin crawl. By 1:45 PM, his shirt was soaked with sweat, his hands were shaking, and he couldn't form coherent thoughts about the financial analysis he'd spent three weeks perfecting.

Alex's sensory overwhelm had nothing to do with presentation anxiety or lack of preparation. The environment itself was attacking his nervous system, making it impossible to access his considerable expertise or communicate effectively. Three months later, after implementing targeted sensory management strategies, Alex delivered the same type of presentation with confidence and clarity, earning recognition for his analytical insights and communication skills.

Open Office Survival Strategies

Modern open office environments present unique challenges for autistic professionals because they maximize exactly the sensory inputs that overwhelm autistic nervous systems. However, specific strategies can transform these challenging spaces into manageable work environments.

Acoustic management becomes essential in environments designed for collaboration but devastating for concentration. Open offices typically generate 50-60 decibels of background noise—enough to significantly impact focus for noise-sensitive individuals while remaining below most people's conscious awareness.

Noise-canceling headphones provide immediate relief from background chatter, HVAC systems, and equipment noise. Choose models that offer both active noise cancellation and comfortable extended wear. Many organizations approve headphones as standard equipment once managers understand their productivity benefits.

Jennifer, a 38-year-old data analyst, increased her accuracy rate by 23% and reduced task completion time by 15% after implementing noise-canceling headphones. Her manager initially worried about her accessibility for quick questions but discovered that scheduled check-ins produced better communication than random interruptions.

White noise or nature sounds can mask unpredictable office noises that trigger startle responses or concentration breaks. Apps providing consistent soundscapes help your brain filter environmental audio more effectively than silence interrupted by sudden sounds.

Strategic seating selection minimizes exposure to high-traffic areas, direct sightlines to movement, and proximity to noisy equipment. Request desk placement near walls, in corners, or away from main walkways. Face your monitor away from movement patterns that create peripheral distractions.

Visual barrier creation using desktop plants, file organizers, or privacy screens reduces peripheral movement detection that can fragment concentration. Your brain processes visual changes automatically, so reducing unnecessary visual input preserves cognitive resources for work tasks.

Lighting optimization addresses one of the most pervasive sensory challenges in office environments. Fluorescent lights flicker at 60 Hz—a frequency that many autistic individuals detect consciously, creating eye strain, headaches, and concentration difficulties.

Desk lamp solutions provide alternative lighting that reduces dependence on overhead fluorescents. Full-spectrum LED desk lamps offer adjustable brightness and color temperature that you can modify throughout the day to match your sensory needs and energy levels.

Monitor positioning prevents glare from windows or overhead lights that can trigger sensory discomfort. Anti-glare screen protectors reduce reflections while blue light filtering glasses minimize harsh LED wavelengths that contribute to eye strain and headaches.

Mark, a 41-year-old software developer, eliminated his daily 3:00 PM headaches by repositioning his monitor to avoid window glare and adding a warm-light desk lamp. These simple changes improved his afternoon productivity by 40% and eliminated the fatigue that previously persisted into evening hours.

Meeting Room Modifications

Conference rooms concentrate multiple sensory challenges while demanding peak cognitive performance for important business discussions. Strategic preparation and environmental modifications help you contribute effectively without sensory overwhelm compromising your participation.

Pre-meeting environmental assessment allows you to identify and address sensory challenges before they impact your performance. Arrive early to adjust lighting, seating, and room setup when possible. Many meeting rooms have individual controls for overhead lights, temperature, and seating arrangements.

Seating strategy development helps you choose positions that minimize sensory input while maximizing your contribution ability. Seats with wall backing reduce stimulation from behind, while positions allowing easy exit access provide psychological comfort that reduces anxiety about being trapped in overwhelming situations.

Lighting modification techniques address the harsh fluorescents common in conference rooms. Request permission to turn off overhead lights when natural light is sufficient, or suggest adjusting blinds to reduce glare. Many modern conference rooms have dimmer controls that few people use but can significantly improve sensory comfort.

Temperature and airflow management becomes critical in crowded meeting spaces where HVAC systems work harder and body heat accumulates. Choose seating away from direct vent airflow and bring layers to adjust your personal temperature without affecting others' comfort.

Audio considerations in meeting rooms include managing echo, speaker volume, and multiple conversation streams. Sit closer to primary speakers to improve audio clarity while reducing background noise. Request that only one person speak at a time during complex discussions.

Sarah, a 35-year-old marketing manager, transformed her meeting participation by requesting agenda items in advance and arriving ten minutes early to adjust the environment. She could then focus on content contribution rather than sensory management during discussions.

Technology accommodations can reduce sensory demands while improving meeting effectiveness. Request written meeting summaries, digital note-sharing, or recorded sessions that allow you to review complex information at your optimal processing pace.

Break management during long meetings prevents sensory accumulation that can trigger overwhelm. Advocate for scheduled breaks every 90 minutes or request permission to step out briefly when sensory load becomes problematic.

Travel and Conference Accommodations

Business travel and professional conferences combine multiple sensory challenges with unfamiliar environments and disrupted routines. Strategic planning and proactive accommodations help you maintain professional effectiveness while managing autism-related challenges.

Airport and transit strategies address the sensory intensity of travel environments while maintaining schedule adherence. Airports combine crowds, announcements, bright lights, and unpredictable sounds in environments designed for efficiency rather than comfort.

Noise management during travel becomes essential for preventing sensory overload before important meetings or presentations. Invest in high-quality noise-canceling headphones and download calming audio content for use during flights, train rides, or hotel stays.

Hotel accommodation requests can significantly improve your sleep quality and recovery time during business trips.

Request rooms away from elevators, ice machines, and high-traffic areas. Corner rooms typically offer better sound insulation and fewer neighbors.

David, a 43-year-old consultant, discovered that requesting ground-floor hotel rooms eliminated the sensory stress of elevator rides and hallway noise above him. This simple modification improved his sleep quality and next-day presentation effectiveness significantly.

Conference survival planning helps you manage multi-day events that combine networking demands with sensory challenges. Large conferences overwhelm even neurotypical attendees, making preparation essential for autistic professionals.

Quiet space identification at conference venues provides essential recovery areas between sessions. Research venue layouts in advance to locate libraries, outdoor spaces, or quiet corridors where you can decompress without missing networking opportunities.

Session selection strategies prevent overscheduling that leads to sensory overwhelm. Choose fewer sessions with more processing time rather than attempting to attend everything. Quality engagement with select content produces better professional value than surface-level exposure to excessive information.

Networking event modifications allow you to participate in professional relationship building without sensory overload. Arrive early to networking events when crowds are smaller and noise levels are manageable. Focus on one-on-one conversations rather than group discussions.

Technology Solutions for Sensory Management

Modern technology offers sophisticated tools for managing sensory challenges in professional environments. These solutions often provide immediate relief while demonstrating your proactive approach to workplace optimization.

Sound management applications transform your smartphone into a powerful sensory management tool. Apps like Noisli, Brain.fm, or simply white noise generators help mask unpredictable office sounds with consistent, manageable audio backgrounds.

Light therapy devices address the mood and energy impacts of inadequate or poor-quality lighting in office environments. Desktop light therapy lamps provide full-spectrum illumination that can improve focus, reduce seasonal depression, and regulate circadian rhythms disrupted by fluorescent lighting.

Environmental monitoring tools help you identify and track sensory triggers in your workplace. Sound level apps, light meters, and temperature monitors provide objective data about environmental conditions that affect your performance and comfort.

Lisa, a 39-year-old financial analyst, used a sound level app to document that her workspace consistently exceeded 65 decibels during peak hours. This data supported her accommodation request for a quieter office location and demonstrated the business impact of environmental factors on productivity.

Wearable technology solutions provide discreet sensory management that doesn't require environmental modifications. Smartwatches with vibration alerts can replace audible notifications, while fitness trackers monitor stress levels that correlate with sensory overload.

Blue light filtering tools reduce the harsh LED wavelengths common in modern office lighting and computer screens. Software applications like f.lux automatically adjust screen color temperature throughout the day, while blue light filtering glasses provide protection from overhead lighting.

Temperature regulation accessories help you maintain comfort in environments with variable or uncomfortable climate control. Desk fans, heating pads, or wearable cooling devices provide personal temperature management without affecting colleagues.

Organizational software reduces cognitive load by providing external structure for complex information management. Project management apps, calendar systems, and note-taking tools free mental resources for sensory processing and work tasks.

Action Items: Sensory Toolkit Creation

This systematic approach helps you develop a personalized sensory management system that addresses your specific workplace challenges while maintaining professional effectiveness.

Sensory Assessment Phase

1. **Environmental Audit Completion** Document your current workplace sensory challenges:

Acoustic Environment Analysis

- Record typical noise levels throughout your workday using a sound meter app

- Identify specific sounds that trigger distraction or discomfort

- Note correlation between noise levels and concentration ability

- Track how sound changes affect your work quality and completion time

Visual Environment Evaluation

- Assess lighting quality, glare sources, and visual distractions in your workspace

- Document eye strain, headaches, or concentration difficulties related to visual factors

- Identify optimal lighting conditions for different types of work

- Note how lighting changes throughout the day affect your energy and performance

Physical Environment Assessment

- Monitor temperature, airflow, and seating comfort throughout your workday

- Track correlations between physical discomfort and work performance

- Identify optimal environmental conditions for sustained concentration

- Document how environmental factors affect your energy levels and mood

2. **Sensory Trigger Documentation** Create detailed records of specific sensory challenges:

High-Impact Triggers

- List environmental factors that consistently cause distraction or discomfort
- Rate severity of different sensory challenges on a 1-5 scale
- Document how triggers affect your work quality and efficiency
- Identify patterns in trigger exposure and recovery requirements

Medium-Impact Challenges

- Note environmental factors that occasionally affect your performance
- Track circumstances that make moderate triggers more problematic
- Document cumulative effects of multiple moderate triggers
- Identify early warning signs of sensory overload development

Solution Development Phase

3. **Technology Solution Research** Investigate tools that address your specific sensory needs:

Audio Management Tools

- Research noise-canceling headphones within your budget range

- Download and test white noise or nature sound applications
- Explore music or soundscape options that improve your concentration
- Investigate workplace policies regarding headphone use during work hours

Visual Management Solutions

- Research desk lamps that provide full-spectrum or adjustable lighting
- Investigate anti-glare screen protectors and blue light filtering options
- Explore privacy screens or visual barriers for your workspace
- Consider apps that adjust computer screen lighting throughout the day

Environmental Control Options

- Research personal temperature regulation devices suitable for office use
- Investigate air quality monitors or purifiers for your workspace
- Explore ergonomic seating or workspace modifications
- Consider organizational tools that reduce visual clutter and cognitive load

4. **Accommodation Strategy Development** Plan systematic approaches to environmental modifications:

Self-Implemented Solutions

- List modifications you can make independently without supervisor approval
- Identify technology purchases you can make with personal funds
- Plan workspace organization changes within your control
- Develop routines that optimize your interaction with current environment

Supervisor Discussion Items

- Prepare requests for environmental modifications requiring approval
- Develop business justifications for accommodation requests
- Research costs and implementation requirements for proposed changes
- Plan presentation of sensory needs as productivity optimization opportunities

Implementation and Testing Phase

5. **Sensory Toolkit Assembly** Build your personalized sensory management system:

Essential Tools Kit

- Noise-canceling headphones or earbuds for audio management

- Desk lamp or lighting modification tools for visual comfort

- Temperature regulation accessories for physical comfort

- Organization tools for reducing cognitive load and visual clutter

Backup and Travel Kit

- Portable versions of essential sensory management tools

- Emergency comfort items for high-stress or overwhelming situations

- Travel-friendly technology solutions for business trips and conferences

- Quick-access items for meeting rooms and unfamiliar environments

6. **Effectiveness Testing Protocol** Systematically evaluate your sensory management solutions:

Baseline Performance Measurement

- Document current work performance metrics before implementing solutions

- Track energy levels, concentration ability, and task completion rates

- Note frequency and severity of sensory overwhelm episodes

- Record end-of-day fatigue levels and recovery time requirements

Solution Impact Assessment

- Test individual solutions separately to identify most effective tools

- Document performance improvements with each sensory management strategy

- Track reduction in sensory overwhelm frequency and severity

- Monitor energy conservation and improved sustainability throughout workdays

Optimization and Maintenance Phase

7. **Continuous Improvement Process** Refine your sensory management approach over time:

Regular Effectiveness Reviews

- Monthly assessment of tool effectiveness and need for adjustments

- Seasonal consideration of changing environmental factors

- Technology updates and new solution research

- Accommodation success evaluation and potential expansion

Professional Integration Strategy

- Communication with colleagues about sensory management needs

- Integration of sensory tools into professional image and workflow

- Advocacy for team-wide environmental improvements that benefit everyone

- Mentoring other professionals with similar sensory challenges

Professional Sensory Management as Competitive Advantage

Effective sensory management transforms potential workplace challenges into demonstrations of self-awareness, strategic planning, and professional optimization. Your systematic approach to environmental factors often produces insights and improvements that benefit entire teams or organizations.

Productivity optimization through sensory management often exceeds accommodation costs within weeks of implementation. Organizations increasingly recognize that environmental modifications supporting neurodivergent employees improve conditions for everyone, creating more comfortable and productive workspaces.

Professional credibility grows when colleagues see your thoughtful approach to workplace effectiveness and your willingness to invest in optimal performance. Your sensory management strategies demonstrate commitment to professional excellence rather than personal limitation.

Leadership opportunities emerge when you help organizations understand how environmental factors affect all employees' performance. Your expertise in sensory management often positions you as a resource for workplace improvement initiatives and accommodation implementation.

The Strategic Framework for Sensory Success

- Open office challenges require systematic approaches to acoustic, visual, and environmental management

- Meeting room modifications enable full participation in important professional discussions without sensory overwhelm

- Travel and conference accommodations maintain professional effectiveness during high-stress business activities

- Technology solutions provide immediate relief while demonstrating proactive workplace optimization

- Systematic sensory toolkit development creates sustainable management strategies that improve long-term career satisfaction

Your mastery of sensory challenges provides the foundation for authentic professional communication that showcases your autism strengths while managing potential difficulties. You're ready to develop communication strategies that transform your directness and systematic thinking into professional advantages.

Chapter 8: Communication Strategies for Autistic Professionals

The feedback from Mark's 360-degree review was consistent across all respondents: "Brilliant analytical mind, but communication needs work." His colleagues appreciated his thorough reports and innovative solutions but found his direct questions "intimidating" and his detailed explanations "overwhelming." His manager suggested communication training to help him develop "softer" interpersonal skills.

Six months later, after understanding his autism diagnosis and developing strategic communication approaches, Mark received feedback describing him as "refreshingly clear and direct" with "exceptional ability to explain complex concepts." The difference wasn't that Mark had changed his fundamental communication style—he'd learned to position his autistic communication patterns as professional strengths while making minor adjustments that improved collaborative effectiveness.

Email vs. Verbal Communication Preferences

Your autism affects how you process and respond to different communication formats, creating natural preferences that can become professional advantages when strategically leveraged. Understanding these patterns allows you to advocate for communication methods that showcase your thinking while meeting workplace collaboration requirements.

Written communication advantages align naturally with autistic information processing patterns. Email, documentation, and written reports allow processing time that verbal communication often doesn't provide. You can organize thoughts systematically, review for accuracy, and provide thorough analysis without the pressure of immediate verbal response.

Processing time benefits in written communication eliminate the stress of rapid-fire conversations that don't match your thinking pace. Complex business decisions often benefit from the careful analysis that written communication enables, even when workplace culture favors quick verbal exchanges.

Consider Sarah, a 37-year-old project manager who transformed team communication by implementing "email before meetings" protocols. Team members sent questions and concerns via email before weekly meetings, allowing Sarah to prepare thorough responses and use meeting time for collaborative discussion rather than information gathering. Team satisfaction increased by 40% because meetings became more focused and productive (3).

Documentation accuracy improves when you can review and refine written communication before sending. Your natural attention to detail becomes a communication asset when you have time to ensure clarity, accuracy, and completeness in important business correspondence.

Reference value of written communication provides permanent records that support project management, decision tracking, and accountability maintenance. Your preference for written communication often improves organizational record-keeping and reduces misunderstandings that arise from verbal-only discussions.

Verbal communication challenges often stem from processing speed differences rather than communication ability. Your systematic thinking produces excellent insights but may require more processing time than typical workplace conversations allow.

Meeting participation optimization requires strategies that work with your processing style rather than against it. Request agenda items in advance when possible, and don't hesitate to ask for clarification time during complex discussions. Your thoughtful responses often provide more value than quick reactions.

Phone conversation management can be particularly challenging because it eliminates visual cues while maintaining pressure for immediate responses. When possible, suggest video calls that provide visual context or follow phone discussions with written summaries that confirm understanding.

Managing Meeting Participation and Social Expectations

Professional meetings combine multiple autism challenges: unpredictable social dynamics, sensory overload potential, and pressure for spontaneous contribution. Strategic approaches help you participate effectively while leveraging your analytical strengths.

Preparation strategies transform meeting challenges into opportunities to showcase your systematic thinking. Review agenda items in advance, prepare questions and comments, and research topics that will be discussed. This preparation allows you to contribute meaningfully without relying on spontaneous verbal processing.

Contribution timing matters more for autistic professionals than neurotypical colleagues. Your most valuable insights often come after processing discussion content rather than during rapid brainstorming phases. Advocate for follow-up opportunities to provide detailed analysis or written input after meetings.

David, a 42-year-old operations analyst, increased his meeting effectiveness by requesting 24-hour response windows for complex decisions. His follow-up emails with detailed analysis became highly valued by his team because they provided thorough consideration of factors that others missed during real-time discussions.

Question strategies help you gather necessary information while respecting meeting flow and social expectations. Prepare clarifying questions in advance, and don't apologize for requesting specific details or concrete examples that help you understand abstract concepts.

Social navigation techniques acknowledge that meetings involve relationship dynamics alongside business content. Your direct communication style can become an asset when positioned as efficiency and clarity rather than social insensitivity.

Energy management during meetings prevents the fatigue that can compromise your contribution quality. Take notes to maintain focus, request breaks during long sessions, and position yourself to minimize sensory distractions that fragment your attention.

Follow-up protocols ensure that your processing time contributes to team outcomes. Offer to provide written analysis after meetings, summarize action items for team distribution, or prepare detailed implementation plans that build on meeting discussions.

Direct Communication in Diplomatic Contexts

Your natural tendency toward direct, clear communication can become a significant professional asset when framed appropriately for business contexts. The key is positioning directness as efficiency and clarity rather than social insensitivity.

Clarity as professionalism reframes your direct communication style as business-focused efficiency. Many organizations value clear, straightforward communication that eliminates ambiguity and reduces misunderstandings. Your autism traits support this communication effectiveness.

Question framing techniques help you gather necessary information while respecting social expectations. Instead of "That doesn't make sense," try "Could you help me understand the connection between X and Y?" This approach seeks the same clarification while acknowledging that understanding might be your responsibility rather than the speaker's failure.

Feedback delivery strategies allow you to provide honest, helpful input while maintaining positive relationships. Focus feedback on specific behaviors or outcomes rather than personal characteristics, and include concrete suggestions for improvement alongside problem identification.

Jennifer, a 38-year-old marketing director, became known for "constructive directness" that helped teams identify and solve problems quickly. She learned to preface direct feedback with context: "I want to help us succeed, so I'd like to point out a potential issue with our timeline." This framing positioned her directness as team support rather than criticism.

Diplomatic language adaptation doesn't require changing your message but can modify delivery methods that improve reception. Adding phrases like "In my analysis" or "From a systematic perspective" provides context for your direct observations while maintaining their clarity and value.

Cultural context awareness helps you adjust communication style for different business situations without compromising your authentic voice. Client presentations might require more diplomatic language than internal team discussions, but your core analytical insights remain valuable in both contexts.

Boundary communication allows you to maintain professional relationships while respecting your autism needs. Clear, direct communication about your preferences often works better than indirect hints that others might misinterpret.

Handling Feedback and Performance Reviews

Performance feedback conversations combine several autism challenges: social interaction pressure, potential criticism processing, and requirements for immediate verbal response. Strategic preparation helps you navigate these important career discussions effectively.

Preparation protocols for performance reviews reduce anxiety while ensuring you can advocate effectively for your contributions and development needs. Review your accomplishments, prepare examples of your impact, and identify areas where you want feedback or support.

Feedback processing strategies acknowledge that you might need time to understand and respond to performance input. Ask for written feedback summaries when possible, and don't hesitate to request follow-up meetings if you need processing time for complex performance discussions.

Self-advocacy techniques help you communicate your value while addressing any performance concerns. Prepare concrete examples of your contributions, and connect your work style to business benefits rather than apologizing for differences.

Mark, a 39-year-old financial analyst, transformed his performance reviews by preparing detailed documentation of his contributions with quantified business impact. His systematic approach to self-evaluation impressed supervisors and led to recognition for analytical excellence and thorough project management.

Improvement area discussion requires balancing honest self-assessment with strategic career positioning. When supervisors identify development areas, focus on specific skills or strategies rather than fundamental personality changes that would compromise your authentic strengths.

Goal setting collaboration ensures that your development plans work with your autism strengths rather than against them. Advocate for goals that leverage your systematic thinking and attention to detail while providing support for areas that challenge your autism traits.

Documentation and follow-up help you track performance feedback implementation and demonstrate your commitment to professional growth. Written summaries of feedback discussions protect your interests while showing proactive engagement with development opportunities.

Action Items: Communication Preference Documentation

This systematic approach helps you identify your optimal communication patterns and develop strategies for professional communication that leverage your autism strengths.

Communication Pattern Analysis

1. **Format Preference Assessment** Document your effectiveness with different communication types:

Written Communication Evaluation

- Track your performance and comfort level with email correspondence
- Note how written format affects your ability to express complex ideas clearly
- Document time requirements for written vs. verbal communication
- Assess quality differences between your written and verbal communication

Verbal Communication Analysis

- Rate your effectiveness in different verbal communication situations
- Note processing time needs for verbal responses in various contexts

- Track energy costs of different types of verbal interaction
- Identify verbal communication situations that showcase vs. challenge your abilities

Meeting Participation Assessment

- Document your contribution quality in different meeting formats
- Track how meeting preparation affects your participation effectiveness
- Note optimal meeting sizes and structures for your contribution style
- Assess how meeting frequency affects your overall communication energy

2. **Processing Style Documentation** Understand your natural communication processing patterns:

Response Time Requirements

- Note situations where you need additional processing time
- Track how processing time affects your response quality and accuracy
- Document optimal response timing for different types of communication
- Identify ways to request processing time professionally

Information Organization Preferences

- Assess how you best organize complex information for communication
- Note formats that help you present systematic analysis effectively
- Track which communication structures showcase your thinking most clearly
- Document preparation methods that optimize your communication effectiveness

Professional Communication Strategy Development

3. **Workplace Communication Optimization** Develop strategies that leverage your communication strengths:

Email Strategy Framework

- Create templates for common business communication types
- Develop systems for organizing and tracking important correspondence
- Plan strategies for using email to prepare for verbal communication
- Design follow-up protocols that reinforce verbal discussions with written summaries

Meeting Participation Enhancement

- Develop preparation protocols for different types of meetings
- Create question frameworks that help you gather necessary information

- Plan contribution strategies that showcase your analytical strengths
- Design follow-up methods for providing detailed analysis after meetings

Feedback Communication Planning

- Prepare frameworks for discussing your communication preferences professionally
- Develop scripts for requesting accommodation in communication format or timing
- Plan strategies for positioning your communication style as business asset
- Create methods for demonstrating communication effectiveness through results

4. **Professional Positioning Strategy** Frame your communication patterns as professional strengths:

Directness as Efficiency

- Develop language that positions clear communication as business benefit
- Create examples demonstrating how direct communication improves outcomes
- Plan strategies for maintaining directness while respecting social expectations
- Prepare responses to feedback about communication style that reinforces value

Systematic Analysis as Expertise

- Document how your thorough communication approach prevents problems
- Create examples of how detailed communication improves project outcomes
- Develop methods for presenting systematic analysis accessibly
- Plan ways to position thoroughness as quality control and risk management

Implementation and Monitoring

5. **Communication Strategy Implementation** Put your communication optimization strategies into practice:

Daily Communication Practice

- Implement preferred communication formats when possible
- Practice positioning your communication style positively
- Use preparation strategies for important communication situations
- Apply energy management techniques for communication-intensive days

Professional Relationship Building

- Communicate your preferences to colleagues and supervisors appropriately
- Demonstrate how your communication style benefits team outcomes

- o Build relationships based on communication effectiveness rather than social performance
- o Seek mentors and colleagues who appreciate direct, thorough communication

6. **Effectiveness Monitoring and Adjustment** Track your communication strategy success and refine approaches:

Communication Outcome Assessment

- o Monitor how communication strategies affect your professional relationships
- o Track whether colleagues and supervisors respond positively to your approach
- o Assess impact on work quality and team collaboration
- o Document career advancement correlation with communication strategy implementation

Continuous Communication Improvement

- o Identify communication strategies that work best in your specific work environment
- o Adjust approaches based on feedback and outcome measurement
- o Seek professional development opportunities that build on your communication strengths
- o Mentor other professionals who could benefit from direct, systematic communication approaches

The Strategic Communication Advantage

Your autism-influenced communication patterns aren't obstacles to overcome—they're professional assets to leverage strategically. Many organizations desperately need the clarity, thoroughness, and analytical depth that your communication style provides, even when initial reactions suggest preference for more conventional approaches.

Business value creation through authentic communication often exceeds the comfort benefits of masking your natural style. Colleagues and clients frequently appreciate directness and clarity once they understand its value, especially in complex business situations where ambiguity creates problems.

Professional differentiation emerges when your communication style becomes associated with quality analysis, clear thinking, and reliable information. Your reputation for thorough, accurate communication becomes a career asset that opens opportunities and builds trust.

Leadership development builds on your natural communication strengths rather than forcing neurotypical leadership styles. Many successful leaders are valued for their clear, direct communication and systematic approach to complex problems—qualities that align naturally with autism traits.

The Foundation for Professional Excellence

- Written communication preferences align with autism processing patterns and often produce superior business outcomes

- Meeting participation optimization showcases analytical strengths while managing social and sensory challenges

- Direct communication becomes a professional asset when positioned as efficiency and clarity

- Feedback handling strategies protect your interests while demonstrating commitment to professional growth

- Systematic communication preference documentation enables strategic advocacy for optimal professional interaction

Your communication mastery provides the foundation for building sustainable work routines that prevent overwhelm while maximizing your professional effectiveness. You're ready to develop systematic approaches to energy management and routine optimization that support long-term career success.

Chapter 9: Building Sustainable Work Routines

The afternoon meltdown happened in the supply closet on a Tuesday. Emma, a 34-year-old project coordinator, had managed to hold herself together through the morning's crisis meeting, the unscheduled client call, the sudden deadline change, and the team lunch that replaced her usual quiet recovery time. But when the printer ran out of toner and she couldn't find replacement cartridges in their usual location, her carefully managed composure collapsed into overwhelming tears and frustration.

Three months later, after implementing systematic routine structures and energy management protocols, Emma handled a similar chaotic day with calm effectiveness. She'd learned that autism requires different work rhythm management than neurotypical approaches, and that building sustainability into her routines prevented the crashes that had previously compromised both her performance and well-being.

Creating Structure in Unstructured Environments

Modern workplaces often operate with minimal structure, expecting employees to adapt fluidly to changing priorities, interruptions, and ambiguous expectations. Your autistic brain thrives with clear structure and predictable patterns, making it essential to create personal organization systems that provide stability within chaotic environments.

Routine development provides the framework that allows your brain to function optimally while maintaining the flexibility that workplace demands require. Effective routines balance your need for predictability with organizational requirements for adaptability.

Morning startup protocols establish consistent beginnings that prepare your nervous system for productive workdays. Your morning routine might include reviewing daily schedules, organizing workspace, and completing preparatory tasks that create mental readiness for the day's challenges.

Consider Michael, a 41-year-old software developer who transformed his productivity by implementing a 30-minute morning routine: reviewing project status, organizing his task list, adjusting his workspace environment, and setting daily priorities. This consistent startup sequence improved his focus and reduced decision fatigue throughout the day.

Priority organization systems help you manage multiple competing demands without becoming overwhelmed by choice paralysis. Your systematic thinking works best when tasks are clearly categorized and sequenced according to logical criteria rather than emotional urgency.

Time blocking strategies create structure within your daily schedule while preserving flexibility for unexpected demands. Dedicate specific time blocks for different types of work—deep analysis, communication, administrative tasks—rather than mixing activities randomly throughout the day.

Transition protocols between different activities or locations help your brain adjust to changing contexts without losing momentum or becoming overwhelmed. Brief transition rituals provide closure for completed tasks while preparing your mind for new activities.

End-of-day closure routines ensure that work stress doesn't carry over into personal time while preparing for the next day's success. Your closure routine might include task documentation, workspace organization, and next-day preparation that provides psychological completion.

Managing Transitions and Interruptions

Workplace interruptions and unexpected transitions create particular challenges for autistic professionals because they disrupt the systematic thinking patterns that support your optimal performance. Strategic approaches help you maintain productivity while accommodating organizational needs for flexibility and responsiveness.

Interruption management requires systems that protect your deep work time while maintaining professional accessibility and collaboration. Complete interruption elimination isn't realistic in most workplaces, but strategic management reduces their impact on your performance and energy.

Signal systems communicate your availability status to colleagues without requiring constant verbal explanation. Simple indicators like closed office doors, headphones, or desk signs can reduce interruptions during focused work periods while maintaining approachable relationships.

Batching strategies group similar activities together to minimize task-switching overhead that depletes your cognitive resources. Dedicate specific times for email responses, phone calls, or administrative tasks rather than handling them sporadically throughout the day.

Sarah, a 36-year-old marketing analyst, increased her daily productivity by 45% through batching communication tasks into two 30-minute periods rather than responding to messages throughout the day. This approach preserved her concentration for analytical work while ensuring timely responses to colleagues and clients.

Context switching protocols provide systematic approaches for transitioning between different types of work without losing momentum or becoming overwhelmed. Brief transition rituals help your brain adjust to new contexts while maintaining optimal performance.

Buffer time planning includes recovery periods between demanding activities that prevent cognitive overload from accumulating throughout the day. Short breaks between complex tasks or social interactions provide essential processing time that maintains your effectiveness.

Flexible structure development creates routine frameworks that can accommodate workplace unpredictability without causing system breakdown. Your structure should provide stability while allowing modification for legitimate business needs.

Energy Management Throughout the Workday

Autistic professionals experience different energy patterns than neurotypical colleagues, particularly regarding social interaction, sensory processing, and masking demands. Understanding and managing these patterns prevents the energy depletion that leads to performance decline and eventual burnout.

Energy monitoring helps you recognize the early signs of depletion before they compromise your work quality or well-being. Your energy levels fluctuate based on task types, environmental factors, and social demands rather than simply time of day.

Peak performance identification reveals when your energy levels naturally support different types of work. You might excel at analytical tasks during morning hours while finding social interactions more manageable in afternoon periods when your initial energy reserves have stabilized.

Energy allocation strategies ensure that your limited resources are directed toward your most important work rather than depleted by low-value activities. Prioritize high-energy tasks during your peak periods while scheduling routine activities during lower-energy times.

David, a 43-year-old financial planner, discovered that his complex analysis work was most effective between 9:00 AM and 11:00 AM, while client meetings were more successful after 2:00 PM when his initial energy had settled into sustainable patterns. Aligning task timing with energy patterns improved both his work quality and job satisfaction.

Recovery protocols provide systematic approaches for restoring energy during the workday rather than allowing depletion to accumulate. Brief recovery periods prevent minor fatigue from developing into major overwhelm that requires extended recovery time.

Social energy budgeting acknowledges that workplace social interactions consume different amounts of energy depending on their type, duration, and participants. Budget your social energy strategically for the most important interactions while minimizing unnecessary social demands.

Masking energy conservation reduces the energy costs of performing neurotypicality by identifying where authenticity is possible and acceptable. Every reduction in masking energy preserves resources for actual work performance and quality contribution.

Preventing Overwhelm and Meltdowns at Work

Workplace overwhelm and potential meltdowns represent the endpoint of accumulated stress, sensory overload, and energy depletion that wasn't addressed through preventive strategies. Early recognition and intervention prevent these crisis situations while maintaining your professional reputation and effectiveness.

Early warning recognition helps you identify the subtle signs that overwhelm is developing before it reaches crisis levels. Your early warning signs might include increased irritability, difficulty concentrating, physical tension, or reduced ability to process information effectively.

Escalation interruption provides specific strategies for halting overwhelm progression when early warning signs appear. These interventions might include brief environmental changes, sensory regulation techniques, or temporary activity modifications that prevent crisis development.

Environmental assessment during overwhelm helps you identify and address the specific factors contributing to stress accumulation. Sensory overload, social demands, or cognitive complexity might be creating overwhelm that environmental modifications can address.

Lisa, a 38-year-old research coordinator, prevented weekly overwhelm episodes by implementing a "stress check" protocol every two hours. When her stress rating exceeded 6 out of 10, she took a five-minute walk outside or practiced brief breathing exercises that reset her nervous system before overwhelm developed.

Crisis management planning provides specific protocols for handling overwhelm if prevention strategies aren't sufficient. Having predetermined plans reduces the additional stress of decision-making during overwhelm while ensuring professional and safe crisis management.

Recovery strategies help you restore equilibrium after overwhelming experiences without extending the recovery time unnecessarily. Systematic recovery approaches return you to optimal function more quickly than unstructured rest periods.

Professional communication about overwhelm needs ensures that colleagues understand your self-regulation strategies without viewing them as performance deficits. Frame your overwhelm prevention as productivity optimization rather than personal limitation.

Action Items: Daily Routine Optimization Plan

This systematic approach helps you develop personalized work routines that leverage your autism strengths while managing energy demands and preventing overwhelm.

Current Pattern Analysis

1. **Energy and Performance Tracking** Monitor your natural patterns for one full week:

Hourly Energy Assessment

- Rate your energy level every hour on a 1-10 scale

- Note what types of activities preceded high and low energy periods
- Track correlation between specific tasks and energy changes
- Document time periods when you feel most and least effective

Task Performance Correlation

- Record which types of work feel easiest at different times
- Note when complex analysis, communication, or administrative tasks work best
- Track quality differences in work completed at various energy levels
- Document how task sequence affects your overall daily performance

Overwhelm Pattern Documentation

- Identify situations, times, or circumstances that consistently create stress
- Track early warning signs that precede overwhelm or fatigue
- Note environmental factors that contribute to overwhelm development
- Document recovery requirements after stressful periods

2. **Current Routine Effectiveness Evaluation** Assess how your existing routines support or hinder optimal performance:

Structure vs. Flexibility Balance

- Evaluate how much structure you currently have in your workday
- Note areas where more structure would improve performance
- Identify flexibility requirements that must be accommodated
- Assess how current routines handle unexpected changes or interruptions

Transition Management Assessment

- Document how you currently handle task switching and context changes
- Note which transitions feel smooth vs. difficult or draining
- Track time required to regain focus after interruptions
- Evaluate effectiveness of current transition strategies

Optimal Routine Design

3. **Peak Performance Schedule Development** Design daily routines that align with your natural energy patterns:

Morning Routine Protocol

- Develop consistent morning startup sequence that prepares you for productive work

- Include workspace organization, priority setting, and environmental optimization

- Plan for reviewing daily schedules and identifying potential challenges

- Build in brief mindfulness or centering activity that establishes calm focus

Energy-Task Alignment Planning

- Schedule your most demanding analytical work during peak energy periods

- Plan communication and social tasks during times when interaction feels more manageable

- Reserve routine administrative work for lower-energy periods

- Build recovery time after energy-intensive activities

End-of-Day Closure Design

- Create systematic closure routine that provides psychological completion

- Include documentation of completed work and next-day preparation

- Plan workspace organization that supports next-day startup

- Build in transition activity that separates work from personal time

4. **Interruption and Flexibility Management System** Develop approaches that protect your productivity while accommodating workplace needs:

Interruption Protection Strategies

- Establish specific "deep work" periods with minimal interruption availability

- Create communication protocols that batch non-urgent requests

- Develop signal systems that indicate your availability status to colleagues

- Plan alternative communication methods for urgent needs during focus time

Flexible Structure Framework

- Design routine templates that can accommodate schedule changes

- Create backup plans for when primary routines are disrupted

- Develop rapid reorganization strategies for unexpected priority changes

- Build buffer time into schedules to absorb minor disruptions without stress

Energy Management Implementation

5. **Daily Energy Budget Planning** Allocate your energy resources strategically throughout the workday:

High-Energy Activity Planning

- Schedule complex analysis, important presentations, or challenging projects during peak energy periods
- Limit high-energy activities to sustainable quantities based on your capacity
- Plan recovery time after energy-intensive work to prevent accumulation of fatigue
- Reserve energy buffer for unexpected high-priority demands

Social Energy Management

- Budget specific amounts of social energy for different types of interactions
- Schedule important social interactions (meetings, presentations) during optimal times
- Plan solo work time between social activities to allow energy restoration
- Develop strategies for declining or modifying low-value social demands

Masking Energy Conservation

- Identify workplace situations where authentic self-expression is acceptable
- Reduce unnecessary masking in low-stakes interactions to preserve energy

- Plan higher masking periods strategically around important professional interactions
- Create recovery protocols after periods requiring intensive masking

6. **Overwhelm Prevention System** Implement early intervention strategies that prevent crisis situations:

Warning Sign Monitoring Protocol

- Develop regular check-ins with yourself to assess stress and energy levels
- Create simple rating systems for quickly evaluating your current state
- Identify specific early warning signs that predict overwhelm development
- Plan immediate intervention strategies when warning signs appear

Environmental Management Strategies

- Modify your workspace environment to reduce ongoing sensory stress
- Develop portable sensory management tools for various work locations
- Create backup environmental options when primary workspace becomes overwhelming
- Plan escape routes and quiet spaces for emergency overwhelm management

Crisis Management Planning

- Develop specific protocols for handling overwhelm if prevention fails

- Create professional communication strategies for managing overwhelm at work

- Plan recovery activities that restore equilibrium quickly and effectively

- Establish support systems for crisis situations that maintain professional relationships

Implementation and Optimization

7. **Routine Implementation Strategy** Systematically implement your optimized routines:

Gradual Implementation Planning

- Implement one routine element at a time to avoid overwhelming system changes

- Test routine modifications for at least one week before adding new elements

- Document effectiveness of each routine component separately

- Adjust timing, duration, or content based on real-world testing results

Professional Integration

- Communicate routine needs to supervisors and colleagues appropriately

- Position routine requirements as productivity optimization strategies

- Demonstrate how your routines benefit team effectiveness and work quality
- Seek accommodation for routine elements that require organizational support

8. **Continuous Optimization Process** Refine your routines based on ongoing effectiveness assessment:

Regular Routine Review

- Assess routine effectiveness monthly and adjust based on changing needs
- Evaluate how seasonal changes, workload variations, or role modifications affect optimal routines
- Update routines based on new autism self-awareness or accommodation successes
- Seek feedback from colleagues about how your routines affect collaboration and team effectiveness

Professional Development Integration

- Incorporate routine optimization into professional development planning
- Share successful routine strategies with other neurodivergent professionals
- Advocate for organizational policies that support neurodivergent routine needs
- Develop expertise in workplace routine optimization that could benefit your career advancement

The Sustainable Success Framework

Your optimized work routines create the foundation for long-term career sustainability by working with your autistic brain rather than against it. These systems prevent the energy depletion and overwhelm that threaten both your performance and well-being while showcasing your systematic approach to professional excellence.

Productivity amplification through routine optimization often exceeds the time investment required for system development and maintenance. Colleagues frequently notice improved work quality and consistency that builds your professional reputation while reducing your daily stress.

Professional differentiation emerges when your systematic approach to work organization becomes recognized as a valuable skill that benefits entire teams. Your routine optimization expertise positions you as a resource for workplace effectiveness initiatives.

Career sustainability improves dramatically when your daily work experience aligns with your neurological needs rather than fighting against them. This sustainability enables long-term career growth and satisfaction that masking-based approaches cannot maintain.

Essential Elements for Professional Routine Success

- Structured routines provide stability within chaotic work environments while maintaining required flexibility

- Strategic energy management prevents the depletion that leads to performance decline and overwhelm

- Systematic transition and interruption management preserves productivity while accommodating workplace collaboration needs

- Early overwhelm prevention maintains professional effectiveness while protecting personal well-being

- Personalized routine optimization creates competitive advantages through improved consistency and quality

Your mastery of sustainable work routines completes the foundation for immediate workplace success while preparing you for strategic career advancement that leverages your autism strengths in leadership and professional growth opportunities.

Stepping Forward with Sustainable Excellence

Recognition that your autism requires different routine management than neurotypical approaches marks a fundamental shift from accommodating limitations to optimizing strengths. You're no longer trying to force your brain into incompatible patterns—you're creating work structures that allow your natural capabilities to flourish.

This systematic approach to routine development provides benefits that extend beyond individual performance to team effectiveness and organizational success. Your colleagues benefit from your consistent quality, predictable delivery, and systematic approaches to complex challenges.

The routines you develop become increasingly sophisticated and effective as you gain experience with your specific patterns and needs. This growing expertise in autism-friendly work design positions you for leadership opportunities where your insights about sustainable performance benefit entire organizations.

Core Strategies for Long-Term Success

- Daily routine structure provides the foundation for consistent professional performance while accommodating autism processing needs

- Energy management strategies prevent the depletion cycles that threaten both immediate effectiveness and long-term career sustainability

- Systematic approaches to interruption and transition management preserve productivity while maintaining professional collaboration

- Overwhelm prevention protocols protect both work performance and personal well-being through early intervention strategies

- Continuous routine optimization creates competitive advantages through improved quality, consistency, and professional effectiveness

Your sustainable work routine mastery prepares you for the advanced career strategies that transform autism from accommodation need to professional advantage. You're ready to explore strategic career advancement, leadership development, and long-term professional planning that builds on your authentic strengths rather than masking your differences.

Chapter 10: Authentic Professional Networking

The business card exchange at the quarterly industry mixer felt like a choreographed dance that nobody had taught Marcus the steps to. Around him, 200 professionals seamlessly moved between conversations, laughing at jokes he didn't understand, discussing weekend plans that seemed designed to build rapport rather than share actual information. After 90 minutes of forced small talk and collected business cards he'd never use, Marcus felt more professionally isolated than when he'd arrived.

Eight months later, Marcus had built a network of 47 meaningful professional relationships that directly contributed to his career advancement, led to three consulting opportunities, and provided ongoing support for his professional development. The transformation didn't happen through mastering traditional networking—it came from developing networking strategies that worked with his autistic brain rather than against it.

Networking Strategies That Work for Autistic Brains

Traditional networking approaches assume that relationship building happens through casual social interaction, spontaneous conversation, and broad relationship cultivation. Your autistic brain operates differently, creating opportunities to build professional networks through systematic approaches that often produce deeper, more authentic relationships than conventional methods.

Purpose-driven networking aligns with your systematic thinking by focusing on specific professional objectives rather than general social interaction. Instead of attending events to "meet people," identify particular goals like learning about industry trends, finding mentors in specific areas, or connecting with professionals who share technical interests.

Research-based preparation transforms networking from unpredictable social performance into systematic professional investigation. Before events or meetings, research attendees, speakers, and organizations represented. This preparation provides conversation topics that feel natural and professionally relevant rather than forced social chatter.

Consider Jennifer, a 37-year-old data scientist who revolutionized her networking approach by focusing on industry-specific technical conferences rather than general business events. She prepared by reading speakers' recent publications and identifying specific questions about their methodologies. This preparation led to substantive conversations that developed into ongoing professional relationships and collaboration opportunities.

Structured conversation frameworks provide systematic approaches to professional discussions that feel more natural than random small talk. Develop question sequences that gather information systematically while demonstrating your professional knowledge and interests.

Value-first relationship building establishes connections by offering assistance, information, or expertise rather than seeking immediate benefit. Your systematic approach to problem-solving and analytical thinking often provides genuine value that creates stronger relationship foundations than social bonding attempts.

Follow-up systematization ensures that networking contacts develop into meaningful professional relationships through consistent, professional communication. Your natural preference for clear communication and reliable follow-through becomes a networking asset when systematically applied.

Quality Over Quantity Relationship Building

Your autism naturally aligns with relationship approaches that prioritize depth over breadth, creating opportunities to build professional networks that provide more career value than extensive but superficial contact lists. This focus on quality relationships often produces better professional outcomes while requiring less social energy.

Deep relationship development leverages your systematic thinking to understand colleagues' professional challenges, goals, and expertise areas. These deeper relationships provide mutual support, collaboration opportunities, and career advancement possibilities that superficial networking cannot match.

Specialized network focus concentrates your relationship-building efforts on professionals who share technical interests, industry focus, or career objectives. This specialization makes conversations more natural while creating networks with higher professional relevance and mutual benefit potential.

Sarah, a 35-year-old operations manager, built her career network by focusing exclusively on professionals interested in process optimization and quality management. Her specialized focus led to speaking opportunities, consulting projects, and eventually a promotion to director level when her network recommended her for a position at a partner organization.

Expertise-based positioning establishes your professional value within networks by consistently sharing knowledge, analysis, and problem-solving approaches that demonstrate your capabilities. Your autism strengths in systematic thinking and detailed analysis become networking assets when shared appropriately.

Long-term relationship maintenance uses your natural reliability and consistency to maintain professional connections through regular, professional communication. Your systematic approach to relationship maintenance often outperforms sporadic social interaction in building career-supporting networks.

Mutual benefit focus ensures that professional relationships provide value to both parties rather than one-sided connection attempts. Your analytical thinking helps identify ways to support colleagues' professional objectives while advancing your own career goals.

Industry Events and Conference Survival

Professional conferences and industry events concentrate multiple autism challenges—crowds, noise, unpredictable schedules, and intensive social interaction—while presenting essential networking and professional development opportunities. Strategic approaches help you maximize conference benefits while managing sensory and social demands.

Pre-event planning transforms conferences from overwhelming social chaos into structured professional development opportunities. Review conference schedules, speaker information, and attendee lists to identify specific sessions and networking targets that align with your professional objectives.

Energy management strategies prevent conference burnout by balancing high-energy networking activities with lower-demand professional development sessions. Plan your conference schedule to include recovery time between intensive social interactions and demanding presentations.

Focused attendance planning concentrates your conference energy on activities that provide maximum professional value rather than attempting to attend everything available. Choose fewer sessions with more thorough engagement rather than superficial participation in multiple events.

David, a 42-year-old software architect, improved his conference experience by attending only morning sessions and using afternoons for one-on-one meetings with speakers and industry contacts. This approach reduced sensory overload while enabling deeper professional conversations that produced ongoing collaboration opportunities.

Networking event modification adapts traditional networking formats to your processing style and social needs. Arrive early when crowds are smaller, focus on speaker meet-and-greets rather than general networking periods, and use exhibit halls for structured conversations with vendor representatives.

Information processing optimization helps you absorb and utilize conference content effectively despite potential sensory challenges. Take detailed notes during sessions, request presentation materials when available, and plan post-conference processing time to integrate new information.

Professional presence maintenance ensures that sensory management and social challenges don't compromise your professional reputation or networking effectiveness. Develop strategies for participating authentically while managing autism-related needs discretely and professionally.

Digital Networking Alternatives

Online professional networking platforms and digital communication tools often provide autism-friendly alternatives to traditional face-to-face networking while offering global reach and asynchronous communication benefits that align with your processing preferences.

LinkedIn optimization transforms your professional profile into a networking tool that works continuously rather than requiring constant social performance. Your systematic approach to information organization creates profiles that demonstrate expertise and attract relevant professional connections.

Content sharing strategies establish your professional expertise through systematic sharing of industry analysis, technical insights, and professional commentary. Your natural analytical thinking provides content that attracts quality professional connections while demonstrating your capabilities.

Virtual event participation offers networking opportunities without the sensory challenges of in-person events. Virtual conferences, webinars, and online professional meetings provide access to industry content and networking opportunities with greater environmental control and reduced social pressure.

Lisa, a 38-year-old marketing analyst, built her professional network primarily through LinkedIn content sharing and virtual industry events. Her analytical posts about marketing trends attracted connections with senior marketing executives, leading to speaking opportunities and eventually a director-level position at a Fortune 500 company.

Online community engagement in professional forums, industry groups, and specialized platforms allows you to demonstrate expertise while building relationships through shared professional interests rather than social performance.

Email and messaging relationship building leverages your written communication strengths to develop professional relationships through thoughtful, well-prepared correspondence rather than spontaneous verbal interaction.

Professional portfolio development showcases your systematic work and analytical capabilities through online platforms that allow detailed presentation of your professional achievements and expertise areas.

Action Items: Personalized Networking Plan

This systematic approach helps you develop networking strategies that leverage your autism strengths while building professional relationships that support your career advancement.

Networking Assessment and Goal Setting

1. **Current Network Analysis** Evaluate your existing professional relationships and networking patterns:

Relationship Inventory

- List current professional contacts and categorize by relationship strength

- Assess how current relationships support your career objectives

- Identify gaps in your professional network that limit career advancement

- Evaluate the professional value you currently provide to your network

Networking Strengths and Challenges Assessment

- Document networking activities that feel natural and professionally productive

- Identify networking situations that create stress or require excessive energy

- Assess your current networking results relative to effort invested

- Note specific autism traits that could become networking advantages

2. **Professional Networking Objective Development**
Establish clear goals that guide your relationship-building efforts:

Career Advancement Networking Goals

- Identify specific professionals who could provide mentorship or career guidance

- Determine industry connections needed for career transition or advancement

- Set targets for building relationships with potential collaborators or clients
- Plan networking activities that support specific professional development objectives

Expertise Sharing and Recognition Goals

- Define how you want to be known within your professional community
- Plan strategies for demonstrating your analytical and systematic thinking strengths
- Identify speaking, writing, or consulting opportunities that build professional recognition
- Develop approaches for sharing your autism-related workplace optimization expertise

Strategic Networking Approach Development

3. **Personalized Networking Strategy Design** Create networking approaches that align with your processing style and professional objectives:

Research-Based Networking Framework

- Develop systematic approaches for researching networking targets and opportunities
- Create preparation protocols for networking events and professional meetings
- Plan conversation frameworks that feel natural while gathering professional information

- Design follow-up systems that maintain relationships through consistent professional communication

Value-First Relationship Building Strategy

- Identify ways your analytical thinking and systematic approaches can help other professionals

- Develop strategies for sharing expertise without overwhelming or lecturing contacts

- Plan approaches for offering assistance that builds mutual professional benefit

- Create systems for tracking relationship development and reciprocal value exchange

4. **Event and Platform Strategy Planning** Choose networking venues and platforms that optimize your relationship-building effectiveness:

In-Person Event Strategy

- Identify industry conferences, professional meetings, and events that align with your interests

- Develop preparation protocols for networking events that reduce anxiety and improve effectiveness

- Plan energy management strategies for intensive networking periods

- Create backup plans for networking event overwhelm or social challenges

Digital Networking Platform Optimization

- o Optimize LinkedIn and other professional profiles to attract relevant connections

- o Develop content sharing strategies that demonstrate expertise and attract quality contacts

- o Plan virtual event participation that provides networking opportunities with greater control

- o Create online relationship building approaches that leverage your written communication strengths

Implementation and Relationship Management

5. **Networking Activity Implementation** Execute your networking plan through systematic professional relationship building:

Monthly Networking Activity Planning

- o Schedule specific networking activities that align with your energy and professional schedule

- o Plan preparation time for networking events and professional meetings

- o Balance high-energy networking activities with lower-demand relationship maintenance

- o Track networking activity effectiveness and adjust approaches based on results

Professional Relationship Development Protocol

- Implement systematic follow-up procedures for new professional contacts
- Develop regular communication schedules for maintaining important relationships
- Create value-sharing systems that strengthen professional connections over time
- Plan relationship progression strategies that develop surface contacts into meaningful professional relationships

6. **Network Value Assessment and Optimization** Monitor networking effectiveness and optimize approaches for maximum professional benefit:

Relationship Quality Measurement

- Assess the professional value and mutual benefit of your networking relationships
- Track how networking contacts contribute to your career advancement and professional development
- Evaluate the sustainability of your networking approaches relative to energy investment
- Monitor professional reputation development within your networking communities

Continuous Networking Improvement

- Adjust networking strategies based on what produces the most valuable professional relationships

- Refine networking approaches to align with changing career objectives and professional development

- Expand successful networking strategies while eliminating ineffective relationship building approaches

- Share networking successes with other autistic professionals who could benefit from your approaches

Professional Authenticity in Relationship Building

Your most effective networking happens when you can be authentic about your professional strengths and working style rather than masking your differences to fit traditional networking expectations. This authenticity often attracts higher-quality professional relationships while requiring less energy than performance-based networking.

Systematic thinking as networking strength helps you analyze professional challenges, identify solutions, and provide valuable insights that create meaningful relationship foundations. Your analytical approach to business problems often provides more networking value than social charm or casual relationship building.

Reliable communication patterns become networking assets when consistently applied over time. Your preference for clear, direct communication and systematic follow-through builds trust and professional respect that supports long-term relationship development.

Specialized expertise positioning allows you to build networks around your professional strengths rather than general social interaction. Your depth of knowledge in specific areas attracts professionals who value expertise over broad relationship networks.

The Strategic Networking Foundation

Your networking success builds on authenticity, systematic approaches, and value-focused relationship building rather than traditional social performance. This foundation creates professional networks that provide genuine career support while aligning with your natural communication and relationship patterns.

Professional reputation development through authentic networking often produces stronger career advancement opportunities than broad but superficial relationship networks. Your systematic approach to professional relationships frequently creates deeper connections that provide mutual career benefit over extended periods.

Industry expertise recognition emerges when your networking focuses on sharing knowledge and analytical thinking rather than social relationship building. This expertise-based networking positions you as a valuable professional resource while building relationships based on mutual respect and professional value.

Strategies for Authentic Professional Connection

- Research-based networking preparation transforms unpredictable social interaction into systematic professional investigation

- Quality relationship focus produces deeper professional connections that provide greater career value than broad contact networks

- Strategic conference participation maximizes professional development opportunities while managing sensory and social challenges

- Digital networking platforms provide autism-friendly alternatives that leverage written communication strengths

- Systematic networking plans create sustainable relationship building approaches that align with autism processing patterns

Your authentic networking approach provides the foundation for leadership development that builds on your systematic thinking and analytical strengths rather than requiring neurotypical leadership performance.

Chapter 11: Leadership Through an Autism Lens

The promotion announcement surprised everyone, including Rachel herself. After eight years as a senior analyst, her systematic approach to process improvement and her reputation for clear, honest communication had caught executive attention. But as she prepared for her first team meeting as department manager, Rachel wondered how her autism would affect her ability to lead neurotypical team members who expected very different leadership styles than what came naturally to her.

Eighteen months later, Rachel's team had the highest productivity ratings in the organization, the lowest turnover rate in company history, and had implemented innovative processes that other departments were adopting company-wide. Her success didn't come from learning neurotypical leadership techniques—it came from understanding how her autism traits could become leadership assets when applied strategically and authentically.

Autistic Leadership Strengths and Challenges

Your autism provides distinctive leadership capabilities that often address exactly what modern organizations need but rarely find in traditional leadership approaches. Understanding these strengths—and the challenges they might create—allows you to develop authentic leadership styles that leverage your neurological differences as professional assets.

Systematic decision-making represents one of your strongest leadership capabilities because it ensures that choices are based on thorough analysis rather than impulse, emotion, or organizational politics. Your natural tendency to consider multiple variables and analyze potential consequences produces more thoughtful decisions that serve long-term organizational interests.

Consistent leadership behavior creates team environments where expectations are clear and responses are predictable. Your autism traits naturally resist the mood-based leadership fluctuations that create team anxiety and uncertainty. Team members can depend on consistent feedback, fair treatment, and logical decision-making regardless of external pressures or interpersonal dynamics.

Consider Mark, a 41-year-old engineering manager whose team appreciated his predictable communication style and systematic project management approach. During a company crisis that created widespread leadership chaos, Mark's consistent decision-making and clear communication helped his team maintain productivity while other departments struggled with uncertainty and changing directions.

Data-driven leadership aligns with your natural preference for objective analysis over subjective judgment. Your autism brain processes information systematically, making you naturally inclined toward evidence-based decisions that can be explained and defended. This approach builds team confidence while producing measurable results.

Process optimization expertise stems from your ability to see inefficiencies and systematic improvements that others miss. Your pattern recognition skills identify workflow problems, communication breakdowns, and resource allocation issues that compromise team effectiveness.

These observations often lead to productivity improvements that benefit entire organizations.

Direct communication benefits cut through organizational ambiguity and political maneuvering that confuses team members and wastes time. Your natural tendency toward clear, honest communication helps teams understand expectations, receive useful feedback, and focus on productive work rather than interpreting hidden meanings or navigating social complexities.

Challenge areas require strategic management rather than fundamental personality changes. Your direct communication style might need diplomatic framing for sensitive situations. Your systematic decision-making might require acceleration for time-sensitive choices. Your need for clear information might require patience with ambiguous organizational situations.

Managing Neurotypical Team Members

Leading neurotypical team members requires understanding how their social and communication needs differ from yours while building on shared professional objectives. Your leadership success comes from adapting your approach to team needs rather than expecting team members to adapt to your communication style.

Communication adaptation strategies help you translate your direct, systematic communication into formats that neurotypical team members receive positively. This doesn't mean changing your message but may require adjusting delivery methods to account for social expectations and emotional processing needs.

Social needs recognition acknowledges that your team members might need relationship-building activities, recognition of personal achievements, and casual interaction opportunities that don't feel natural to you but significantly affect their job satisfaction and performance.

Feedback delivery optimization uses your analytical thinking to provide specific, actionable guidance while accounting for neurotypical emotional responses to criticism. Frame feedback in terms of problem-solving and professional development rather than performance deficits or personal shortcomings.

Sarah, a 36-year-old operations director, learned to begin feedback conversations by acknowledging team members' strengths before addressing improvement areas. Her systematic analysis of performance issues remained unchanged, but this framing helped team members receive her insights as development opportunities rather than criticism.

Motivation strategy development recognizes that your team members might be motivated by social recognition, career advancement opportunities, or collaborative achievement rather than the systematic accomplishment that drives your own performance. Understanding these different motivation patterns helps you provide leadership that inspires rather than simply directs.

Meeting facilitation approaches balance your preference for structured, agenda-driven discussions with team members' needs for collaborative input and relationship building. Plan meetings that include both systematic information sharing and opportunities for team interaction and creative input.

Delegation frameworks use your systematic thinking to assign tasks clearly while providing team members the autonomy and flexibility they need for optimal performance. Your detailed planning and clear expectations create structure that supports rather than constrains team effectiveness.

Creating Inclusive Team Environments

Your autism experience with feeling different and requiring accommodations creates natural empathy for team members who need support, flexibility, or non-traditional working arrangements. This understanding often helps you build more inclusive teams than leaders who assume everyone works optimally under standard conditions.

Accommodation awareness helps you recognize when team members might benefit from environmental modifications, communication adjustments, or schedule flexibility. Your understanding of how small changes can dramatically improve performance makes you naturally supportive of requests that might seem unnecessary to other leaders.

Communication style diversity acknowledges that team members process information differently and might need various formats for optimal understanding. Your experience with needing written instructions or processing time helps you provide information in multiple formats that serve different team members' needs.

Strength-based assignments use your analytical thinking to match team members' capabilities with appropriate tasks rather than forcing everyone into identical roles. Your systematic approach to understanding individual strengths often produces more effective team performance than one-size-fits-all task distribution.

David, a 43-year-old project manager, revolutionized his team's effectiveness by analyzing each member's optimal working conditions and task preferences. He discovered that some team members performed best with detailed specifications while others preferred high-level objectives. This individualized approach improved team productivity by 35% while increasing job satisfaction scores.

Performance support systems provide the structure and clarity that help all team members succeed rather than assuming everyone can perform optimally without guidance. Your understanding of how clear expectations and systematic processes improve performance benefits neurotypical team members even when they don't realize they need this support.

Conflict resolution approaches use your direct communication style and systematic thinking to address team problems objectively rather than avoiding difficult conversations or allowing interpersonal issues to compromise work quality.

Professional development focus ensures that team members receive growth opportunities based on their capabilities and interests rather than political considerations or social relationships. Your systematic approach to evaluating performance and potential often identifies development opportunities that other leaders miss.

Decision-Making Processes That Benefit from Autistic Thinking

Your autism provides distinctive decision-making capabilities that often produce superior results compared to conventional leadership approaches. These systematic processes can be adapted to team and organizational contexts while maintaining the analytical rigor that makes them effective.

Information gathering systematization ensures that decisions are based on complete, accurate data rather than assumptions, political considerations, or emotional reactions. Your natural tendency to research thoroughly and consider multiple perspectives produces more informed choices that serve long-term organizational interests.

Risk analysis frameworks use your pattern recognition abilities to identify potential problems and their likelihood before they become critical issues. Your systematic thinking naturally considers various scenarios and their consequences, producing more robust decision-making than approaches based on optimism or limited analysis.

Stakeholder impact assessment applies your analytical thinking to understand how decisions affect different groups within and outside your organization. Your autism experience with being affected by decisions you didn't participate in makes you naturally considerate of broader impact patterns that other leaders might overlook.

Jennifer, a 38-year-old marketing director, used systematic stakeholder analysis to evaluate a proposed product launch strategy. Her analysis identified potential negative impacts on customer service and technical support teams that other leaders had missed. Addressing these concerns before launch prevented customer satisfaction problems and employee overwhelm that could have damaged the company's reputation.

Timeline and resource planning leverages your detail-oriented thinking to ensure that decisions can be implemented effectively with available resources and realistic timeframes. Your systematic approach to project planning often prevents the resource conflicts and timeline problems that compromise decision implementation.

Documentation and communication protocols ensure that decisions are recorded clearly and communicated effectively to all relevant parties. Your preference for clear, detailed communication helps prevent the misunderstandings and inconsistent implementation that often undermine leadership decisions.

Feedback integration systems use your analytical thinking to evaluate decision outcomes and adjust approaches based on results rather than defending choices that aren't working effectively. Your systematic approach to learning from data rather than protecting ego often produces continuous improvement in decision-making quality.

Action Items: Leadership Style Assessment and Development Plan

This systematic approach helps you identify your natural leadership strengths and develop strategies for leading effectively while honoring your authentic autism traits.

Leadership Strengths and Style Assessment

1. **Natural Leadership Pattern Analysis** Document your current leadership approaches and their effectiveness:

Decision-Making Style Documentation

- o Record how you currently make decisions and what information you prioritize
- o Assess the effectiveness of your systematic decision-making approach
- o Note how your decisions are received by team members and supervisors
- o Identify decision-making strengths that could be expanded or better utilized

Communication Leadership Assessment

- o Document your natural communication style and how it affects team dynamics
- o Assess how team members respond to your direct communication approach
- o Note situations where your communication style is most and least effective
- o Identify communication adjustments that might improve team relationships without compromising authenticity

Team Management Approach Evaluation

- o Record how you currently organize work, assign tasks, and monitor progress
- o Assess team member satisfaction with your management style and expectations
- o Note areas where your systematic approach benefits vs. challenges team effectiveness

- Identify management practices that showcase your autism strengths most effectively

2. **Leadership Challenge and Opportunity Identification** Understand areas where autism traits might create leadership challenges or advantages:

Autism-Related Leadership Strengths

- Document systematic thinking applications that benefit team performance

- Identify how your attention to detail and process orientation help teams succeed

- Note reliability and consistency patterns that build team trust and confidence

- Assess how your analytical thinking produces better outcomes than conventional approaches

Leadership Development Areas

- Identify situations where autism traits might create team management challenges

- Note neurotypical team member needs that require adaptation without compromising authenticity

- Assess areas where professional development could enhance leadership effectiveness

- Document feedback from team members about leadership style preferences and needs

Authentic Leadership Development Strategy

3. **Strength-Based Leadership Approach Design**
   Develop leadership methods that leverage autism advantages while meeting team needs:

Systematic Leadership Framework Development

- Create decision-making processes that use your analytical thinking while including team input

- Develop communication approaches that maintain directness while respecting emotional needs

- Design team organization systems that provide structure while allowing individual flexibility

- Plan leadership routines that create predictability while accommodating changing business needs

Team-Centered Adaptation Strategies

- Identify ways to frame your direct communication that team members receive positively

- Develop feedback delivery methods that provide clear guidance while supporting team member confidence

- Create meeting facilitation approaches that balance structure with collaborative input

- Plan motivation strategies that connect individual team member drives with systematic goal achievement

4. **Inclusive Leadership Implementation** Build teams that benefit from diversity while leveraging your autism perspective:

Accommodation and Support System Development

- Create team environments that support different working styles and communication preferences
- Develop policies that provide flexibility while maintaining performance standards
- Design support systems that help all team members succeed regardless of neurotype
- Plan professional development opportunities that build on individual strengths and interests

Conflict Resolution and Problem-Solving Framework

- Develop systematic approaches to team conflicts that address root causes rather than symptoms
- Create communication protocols that prevent misunderstandings while respecting different styles
- Design performance management systems that provide clear expectations and fair evaluation
- Plan team building activities that build collaboration without requiring social performance

Leadership Effectiveness Monitoring and Development

5. **Leadership Impact Assessment Protocol** Measure your leadership effectiveness and refine approaches based on results:

Team Performance and Satisfaction Measurement

- Track team productivity, quality, and achievement metrics under your leadership
- Monitor team member satisfaction, retention, and professional development progress
- Assess how your leadership style affects team collaboration and innovation
- Document feedback from team members about leadership effectiveness and support needs

Personal Leadership Development Tracking

- Monitor your own leadership satisfaction and energy sustainability
- Track professional recognition and advancement opportunities related to leadership performance
- Assess how leadership responsibilities affect your autism management and overall well-being
- Document leadership successes that could be replicated or expanded

6. **Continuous Leadership Improvement Planning** Develop ongoing leadership development that builds on autism strengths while addressing growth areas:

Professional Leadership Development Strategy

- o Identify training opportunities that build on your systematic thinking and analytical strengths

- o Plan mentorship relationships with leaders who appreciate direct communication and data-driven decisions

- o Seek speaking or writing opportunities that share your autism-informed leadership insights

- o Develop expertise in inclusive leadership that could advance your career while helping other professionals

Leadership Legacy and Impact Planning

- o Plan how your autism-informed leadership approach could benefit broader organizational culture

- o Develop strategies for mentoring other neurodivergent professionals in leadership roles

- o Create systems for sharing successful autism leadership practices with other managers

- o Plan career advancement strategies that leverage your unique leadership perspective and capabilities

Building Sustainable Leadership Success

Your autism-informed leadership approach often produces better team outcomes than conventional leadership styles while requiring less energy than masking-based management approaches. This sustainability enables long-term leadership success that benefits both your career advancement and organizational effectiveness.

Team performance improvements under autism-informed leadership frequently exceed those of traditional management approaches because systematic thinking, consistent behavior, and clear communication address team needs that other leadership styles miss or handle inadequately.

Organizational innovation emerges when your different perspective and systematic problem-solving approach identify solutions that conventional thinking overlooks. Your autism traits often produce breakthrough insights that advance organizational effectiveness while building your leadership reputation.

Professional authenticity in leadership roles attracts team members who value clear communication, fair treatment, and systematic decision-making over political maneuvering and social performance. This authenticity often creates more loyal, productive teams than leadership based on charisma or social manipulation.

Leadership Through Authentic Strength

Your autism doesn't limit your leadership potential—it provides distinctive capabilities that modern organizations desperately need but rarely find in traditional leadership development. Your systematic thinking, analytical decision-making, and direct communication style address exactly the leadership gaps that cause team frustration and organizational inefficiency.

Success comes from understanding how to adapt your natural leadership approach to team needs rather than fundamentally changing your autism traits. This adaptation maintains your authentic strengths while building inclusive environments where all team members can contribute optimally.

Professional advancement through autism-informed leadership often exceeds expectations because your approach produces measurable results while building team satisfaction and organizational effectiveness. These outcomes create advancement opportunities that recognize your unique leadership value.

Mentorship opportunities emerge when other professionals recognize your systematic approach to leadership challenges and seek guidance about inclusive management, data-driven decisions, or authentic leadership development. Your expertise becomes a career asset that benefits both your advancement and others' professional growth.

Leadership Principles for Professional Excellence

- Systematic decision-making and consistent leadership behavior create team environments that outperform conventional management approaches

- Authentic communication and clear expectations build team trust while eliminating political ambiguity that wastes time and energy

- Inclusive leadership approaches based on accommodation experience create environments where all team members can contribute optimally

- Data-driven leadership decisions produce sustainable results while building professional credibility and advancement opportunities

- Strength-based leadership development leverages autism advantages while adapting to team needs without compromising authenticity

Chapter 12: Strategic Career Transitions

The job posting seemed perfect: "Senior Data Architect - seeking systematic thinker with attention to detail and strong analytical skills." But as Tom read further, phrases like "dynamic team environment," "fast-paced startup culture," and "extensive client interaction" triggered familiar concerns. After his autism diagnosis six months earlier, he'd learned that job descriptions often hid challenges that could make his life miserable, regardless of salary or title advancement.

Nine months later, Tom was thriving in a role at a different company—one that explicitly valued neurodiversity, offered environmental accommodations, and promoted based on analytical contribution rather than social performance. His career transition success came from systematic evaluation of autism-friendly organizational cultures rather than simply pursuing job titles or compensation increases.

Making the Stay-or-Go Decision Using Autism-Informed Criteria

Career transition decisions for autistic professionals require different evaluation criteria than conventional job change calculations. Your assessment must include factors that neurotypical professionals rarely consider but that significantly affect your performance, energy levels, and long-term career sustainability.

Environmental compatibility assessment evaluates how well your current workplace supports your sensory and organizational needs. This goes beyond basic accommodation provision to include organizational culture, workspace design, and management approaches that either support or hinder your optimal performance.

Masking energy costs in your current role significantly affect job satisfaction and career sustainability. Calculate the daily energy expenditure required for professional performance, social interaction, and environmental adaptation. High masking costs indicate that even successful job performance might not be sustainable long-term.

Professional growth alignment considers how advancement opportunities in your current organization match your autism strengths and career interests. Some organizations provide advancement paths that leverage systematic thinking and analytical skills, while others prioritize social performance and relationship management that might limit your career development.

Consider Sarah, a 38-year-old marketing analyst who received excellent performance reviews but realized her advancement opportunities required extensive client entertainment and networking that drained her energy and compromised her work quality. Her stay-or-go analysis revealed that lateral moves to organizations that valued analytical contribution over social performance would better support her career goals.

Accommodation sustainability evaluates whether your current accommodations will remain effective as your role evolves or organizational changes occur. Some accommodations work well in specific roles but become problematic with increased responsibilities, team management duties, or organizational restructuring.

Organizational stability affects how consistently your autism needs will be supported over time. Leadership changes, budget constraints, or cultural shifts can eliminate accommodations or create environments that become increasingly challenging despite initial compatibility.

Career trajectory analysis examines whether your current path leads toward roles that amplify your autism strengths or require capabilities that consistently challenge your neurological differences. Strategic career planning anticipates these trajectory implications rather than reacting to immediate opportunities.

Industry Analysis for Autism-Friendly Environments

Different industries and organizational types provide varying levels of autism compatibility based on their cultural norms, work structures, and success metrics. Systematic industry analysis helps you identify sectors where your autism traits become professional assets rather than accommodation needs.

Technology sector advantages often align naturally with autism strengths because technical competence typically outweighs social performance in hiring and advancement decisions. Many technology companies explicitly value systematic thinking, attention to detail, and innovative problem-solving approaches that correspond with autism traits (4).

Research and development environments frequently provide autism-compatible work structures including independent projects, clear objective measures, and cultures that value thoroughness over speed. Academic research, pharmaceutical development, and engineering design roles often leverage autism strengths naturally.

Financial analysis and accounting sectors benefit from the systematic thinking and attention to detail that characterize autism strengths. These industries typically provide clear performance metrics, structured work environments, and advancement based on analytical competence rather than social networking.

David, a 41-year-old financial analyst, transitioned from retail banking to investment research specifically because the new environment valued deep analytical thinking over client relationship management. His autism traits that seemed problematic in customer-facing roles became significant assets in research-focused positions.

Government and regulatory organizations often provide structured environments, clear policies, and advancement systems that support autism compatibility. These sectors typically offer environmental stability, accommodation support, and success metrics based on competence rather than political navigation.

Healthcare and social services can provide autism-friendly opportunities in analytical roles like health informatics, research coordination, or systems optimization, even though direct patient care might present social and sensory challenges.

Industry red flags include sectors that prioritize relationship management over technical competence, require extensive travel or unpredictable schedules, or maintain high-pressure sales environments that emphasize social performance over systematic achievement.

Job Searching with Autism Disclosure Considerations

Job search strategies must balance the benefits of early disclosure—finding autism-friendly employers—with the risks of discrimination that can limit opportunities before you can demonstrate your capabilities. Strategic disclosure timing and methods help you identify compatible opportunities while protecting yourself from bias.

Research-based employer identification helps you target organizations with demonstrated neurodiversity support rather than applying broadly and hoping for accommodation acceptance. This approach improves your application efficiency while increasing the likelihood of finding truly supportive work environments.

Company culture evaluation examines organizational values, management approaches, and employee support systems that indicate autism compatibility. Look for companies that emphasize systematic processes, data-driven decisions, and outcomes-based performance evaluation rather than relationship-focused success metrics.

Networking for insider information provides authentic insights about organizational culture that public information doesn't reveal. Connect with current or former employees who can share realistic perspectives about accommodation support, management styles, and day-to-day work environment experiences.

Lisa, a 36-year-old operations manager, used LinkedIn to connect with autism professionals at target companies, gaining insights about accommodation processes and management attitudes that helped her identify truly supportive employers rather than those with superficial diversity policies.

Application strategy development determines how to present your qualifications most effectively while managing disclosure decisions strategically. This might involve highlighting systematic thinking and analytical achievements while avoiding premature disclosure that could trigger bias before interviews.

Interview preparation protocols help you prepare for disability disclosure conversations while ensuring that your capabilities are clearly demonstrated before accommodation discussions begin. This preparation includes developing scripts for disclosure timing and content that maintain professional credibility.

Reference management ensures that your professional references can speak knowledgeably about your autism strengths and accommodation needs without compromising your interview chances through premature or inappropriate disclosure.

Interview Strategies for Autistic Professionals

Job interviews combine multiple autism challenges—unpredictable social interaction, sensory stress, and pressure for immediate verbal responses—while requiring peak performance demonstration. Strategic preparation and interview approaches help you showcase your capabilities while managing autism-related challenges.

Preparation intensification uses your systematic thinking strengths to research interview participants, company challenges, and role requirements thoroughly. This preparation provides conversation topics and question responses that feel natural while demonstrating your analytical capabilities and professional knowledge.

Question framework development helps you prepare structured responses that showcase your systematic thinking while providing the specific examples that interviewers seek. Develop STAR method responses (Situation, Task, Action, Result) that highlight your autism strengths in systematic problem-solving and analytical achievement.

Environmental management involves researching interview locations, requesting specific accommodations if needed, and planning sensory management strategies that maintain your optimal performance. This might include bringing noise-canceling headphones for waiting areas, requesting written follow-up materials, or asking about lighting and seating arrangements.

Consider Mark, a 39-year-old software developer who transformed his interview success by requesting virtual interviews when possible and asking for written position descriptions and interview questions in advance. These accommodations allowed him to prepare thoroughly and showcase his technical expertise without the stress of unpredictable social interaction.

Communication strategy adaptation helps you present your direct communication style as professional efficiency while managing potential interviewer preferences for more diplomatic interaction. Practice framing your analytical observations as business insights rather than criticism of current systems.

Strength positioning techniques ensure that your autism traits are presented as professional assets rather than personal characteristics requiring accommodation. Focus discussion on systematic thinking results, quality improvements, and analytical achievements that demonstrate business value.

Disclosure timing decisions require careful consideration of when and how to discuss autism and accommodation needs during the interview process. Some situations benefit from early disclosure that demonstrates self-awareness and accommodation planning, while others require post-offer disclosure that protects against discrimination.

Follow-up systematization uses your organizational strengths to maintain professional communication throughout the interview process while gathering additional information about role requirements and organizational culture that affects your decision-making.

Negotiating Offers with Accommodation Needs

Job offer negotiations provide opportunities to secure both compensation and accommodations that support your long-term success. Strategic negotiation approaches help you obtain necessary support while maintaining positive relationships with new employers.

Accommodation integration into offer discussions presents your needs as professional optimization requirements rather than special requests that create additional employer burden. Frame accommodations as productivity enhancements that benefit both your performance and organizational outcomes.

Documentation preparation ensures that you can provide specific accommodation descriptions, cost estimates, and business justifications that facilitate employer decision-making. Professional documentation reduces negotiation complexity while demonstrating your systematic approach to workplace optimization.

Prioritization strategy development helps you identify which accommodations are essential versus preferred, allowing negotiation flexibility while ensuring your core needs are met. This prioritization prevents accommodation requests from becoming deal-breakers while securing necessary support.

Jennifer, a 37-year-old project manager, successfully negotiated a comprehensive accommodation package by presenting detailed cost-benefit analysis showing how environmental modifications and communication adjustments would improve her productivity by an estimated 25%. Her systematic approach impressed employers while securing necessary support.

Implementation timeline planning provides realistic expectations for accommodation delivery while ensuring that you can begin work effectively. Some accommodations require equipment purchase or facility modifications that need advance planning and budget allocation.

Performance metric alignment connects your accommodation needs to measurable performance improvements that justify accommodation costs while demonstrating your commitment to organizational success. This approach positions accommodations as business investments rather than employee benefits.

Legal protection documentation ensures that accommodation agreements are properly recorded and legally enforceable while maintaining positive employment relationships. This documentation protects your interests without creating adversarial dynamics with new employers.

Action Items: Career Transition Roadmap

This systematic approach helps you evaluate career change decisions and implement transitions that advance your professional goals while supporting your autism needs.

Current Situation Assessment

1. **Comprehensive Role and Environment Evaluation** Systematically assess your current professional situation:

Job Satisfaction and Performance Analysis

- Rate your current job satisfaction across multiple dimensions including work content, environment, relationships, and growth opportunities

- Document your performance patterns and energy levels throughout typical workdays and weeks

- Assess how your current role utilizes vs. underutilizes your autism strengths

- Identify specific aspects of your current position that support vs. challenge your optimal performance

Accommodation and Support Evaluation

- Document current accommodations and their effectiveness in supporting your performance

- Assess organizational culture and management support for your autism needs

- Evaluate accommodation sustainability as your role or organization changes

- Identify gaps between your optimal work environment and current reality

Career Advancement and Growth Assessment

- Analyze advancement opportunities within your current organization and how they align with your strengths

- Evaluate whether your career trajectory leads toward roles that amplify or minimize your autism advantages

- Assess professional development opportunities and their relevance to your career goals

- Document recognition and reward systems and how they align with your contribution style

2. **Market and Industry Research** Investigate career opportunities that better align with your autism strengths:

Autism-Friendly Industry Identification

- Research industries and sectors known for valuing systematic thinking and analytical skills

- Identify organizations with explicit neurodiversity programs or autism-friendly policies

- Analyze job markets in your geographic area or remote work opportunities

- Evaluate industry trends that might create new opportunities for your skill set

Company Culture and Environment Research

- Research specific organizations' management styles, work environments, and employee support systems

- Identify companies with track records of successful autism accommodation and support

- Analyze organizational values and success metrics to determine autism compatibility

- Connect with current or former employees to gather authentic insights about workplace culture

Strategic Transition Planning

3. **Career Transition Decision Framework** Develop systematic criteria for career change decisions:

Decision Matrix Development

- Create weighted criteria for evaluating career opportunities including autism compatibility factors

- Develop scoring systems that account for both traditional career metrics and autism-specific needs

- Plan decision timelines that allow thorough evaluation without missing opportunities

- Create decision documentation that supports rational choice-making rather than emotional reactions

Risk Assessment and Mitigation Planning

- Identify potential risks associated with career transitions including financial, professional, and personal factors

- Develop contingency plans for transition challenges or unsuccessful career moves

- Plan financial preparation for potential gaps between positions or reduced income during transitions

- Create support systems that provide guidance and assistance during transition stress periods

4. **Job Search Strategy Development** Plan systematic approaches to finding and securing autism-compatible career opportunities:

Application and Networking Strategy

- Develop networking approaches that leverage your systematic thinking and professional expertise

- Create application materials that highlight autism strengths while managing disclosure timing
- Plan job search timelines that allow thorough research and preparation without creating pressure
- Develop follow-up systems that maintain professional communication throughout search processes

Interview and Negotiation Preparation

- Prepare interview strategies that showcase your capabilities while managing autism-related challenges
- Develop accommodation disclosure and negotiation approaches that position needs as professional optimization
- Create documentation and justification materials for accommodation requests
- Plan interview environmental management and communication strategies

Implementation and Success Monitoring

5. **Transition Execution and Adaptation** Implement career transitions systematically while monitoring success and making necessary adjustments:

Onboarding and Integration Planning

- Develop systematic approaches to learning new organizational cultures and expectations

- Plan accommodation implementation and adjustment processes for new work environments

- Create relationship building strategies that establish professional credibility and collaboration

- Design performance tracking systems that demonstrate value while identifying improvement opportunities

Success Measurement and Optimization

- Monitor job satisfaction, performance, and energy levels in new positions

- Track accommodation effectiveness and make adjustments as needed

- Assess career advancement progress and alignment with long-term professional goals

- Document successful transition strategies for future career moves or to help other autistic professionals

6. **Long-Term Career Development Planning** Build on successful transitions to create sustainable career advancement strategies:

Continuous Professional Development

- Identify skill development opportunities that build on autism strengths while addressing professional growth needs

- Plan advanced training or education that supports career advancement while honoring learning style preferences

- Develop expertise areas that position you as a valuable resource within your industry or organization

- Create professional reputation building strategies that highlight your unique contributions and capabilities

Career Legacy and Impact Planning

- Plan how your autism-informed career success can benefit other professionals and organizations

- Develop mentorship or advocacy opportunities that share your transition expertise with others

- Create systems for contributing to autism workplace research or organizational policy development

- Design career advancement strategies that leverage your unique perspective for leadership opportunities

Professional Growth Through Strategic Transitions

Your career transitions succeed when they align with your autism strengths rather than requiring you to overcome neurological differences. This alignment often produces career advancement that exceeds conventional paths while requiring less energy than masking-based professional development.

Market differentiation emerges when your autism traits become recognized professional assets rather than accommodation needs. Organizations increasingly value the systematic thinking, quality focus, and analytical depth that autism provides, creating opportunities for professionals who can demonstrate these capabilities effectively.

Industry leadership develops when your autism-informed approach to professional challenges produces innovations and improvements that benefit entire organizations or sectors. Your different perspective often identifies solutions that conventional thinking misses, positioning you for advanced roles and recognition.

Professional authenticity in career transitions attracts employers who value competence over conformity, creating work environments where your autism becomes a competitive advantage rather than an accommodation requirement.

The Strategic Advantage of Authentic Career Development

Your autism doesn't limit your career options—it clarifies which opportunities will provide sustainable success while advancing your professional goals. Strategic transitions build on this clarity to create career trajectories that leverage your strengths while providing the environmental support you need for optimal performance.

Long-term sustainability improves when career decisions account for autism needs proactively rather than reactively. This sustainability enables career advancement that maintains your well-being while achieving professional objectives that benefit both your development and organizational success.

Professional impact often exceeds expectations when your autism traits are applied to appropriate challenges in supportive environments. Your systematic approach to complex problems frequently produces breakthrough results that advance both your career and organizational effectiveness.

Roadmap for Professional Advancement

- Strategic career evaluation uses autism-informed criteria that predict long-term success rather than short-term opportunities

- Industry analysis identifies sectors where autism traits become professional assets rather than accommodation needs

- Systematic job search approaches balance disclosure considerations with authentic self-presentation that attracts compatible employers

- Interview strategies showcase autism strengths while managing neurological differences that might affect performance evaluation

- Offer negotiation integrates accommodation needs with compensation discussions to secure both financial and environmental support

Your mastery of strategic career transitions provides the foundation for long-term professional success that builds on authentic strengths while creating the environmental support necessary for sustained high performance and career satisfaction.

Building Your Professional Future

Recognition that career transitions require autism-specific evaluation criteria marks a fundamental shift from accommodating limitations to optimizing opportunities. You're no longer limited to making conventional career choices work through accommodation—you're identifying and pursuing opportunities that naturally support your success.

This strategic approach to career development often produces advancement opportunities that exceed traditional paths while requiring less energy than masking-based professional growth. Your systematic thinking and analytical capabilities become career accelerators rather than challenges to overcome.

The transitions you make successfully create templates for future career moves while building professional reputation that attracts autism-friendly opportunities. Your growing expertise in autism-compatible career development becomes both a personal asset and a resource for other professionals navigating similar challenges.

Professional Transition Success Factors

- Systematic evaluation of autism compatibility factors predicts career transition success more accurately than conventional metrics
- Industry research identifies sectors and organizations where autism traits naturally align with success requirements

- Strategic disclosure timing balances authenticity with protection against discrimination during job search processes

- Systematic preparation and environmental management optimize interview performance while showcasing professional capabilities

- Accommodation integration into career negotiations secures necessary support while positioning autism needs as professional optimization opportunities

Your career transition mastery completes the foundation for long-term professional success that transforms autism from accommodation need to competitive advantage, positioning you for continued advancement while building sustainable work environments that support optimal performance and professional fulfillment.

Chapter 13: Preventing and Recovering from Autistic Burnout

The email arrived on a Monday morning: "Due to health reasons, I'll be taking an extended leave of absence." Karen's colleagues were surprised—she'd seemed fine just last week, meeting deadlines and maintaining her usual high standards. But Karen's sudden departure wasn't mysterious to those who understood autistic burnout. The executive assistant had been running on empty for months, masking her exhaustion behind professional competence until her nervous system simply shut down.

Three months later, Karen returned to work with a systematic understanding of her energy patterns and burnout prevention strategies. Her recovery wasn't just about rest—it was about fundamentally restructuring her relationship with work to prevent future crashes while maintaining her professional excellence.

Early Warning Signs Specific to Professional Burnout

Autistic burnout differs significantly from typical work stress because it results from the cumulative neurological load of masking, sensory processing, and social performance rather than simple workload or time pressure. Recognizing these specific warning signs enables early intervention that prevents complete system shutdown.

Masking fatigue escalation appears as increasing difficulty maintaining your professional persona throughout the workday. Tasks that previously required minimal conscious effort—eye contact, small talk, office social interactions—begin demanding significant mental energy. You might notice that maintaining professional appearances becomes exhausting by midday rather than manageable throughout full workdays.

Sensory sensitivity amplification manifests as previously tolerable environmental factors becoming unbearable. Office lighting that you managed comfortably for years suddenly triggers headaches. Background conversations that you filtered successfully begin creating overwhelming distraction. Your sensory tolerance decreases progressively, making normal work environments feel hostile and overwhelming.

Consider Michael, a 41-year-old project manager who noticed that fluorescent lights began causing daily headaches after three years of comfortable tolerance. This sensory sensitivity increase was an early warning sign that his overall nervous system was becoming overloaded, not simply an environmental issue requiring accommodation.

Executive function degradation shows up as increasing difficulty with organization, time management, and task prioritization that were previously manageable. You might find yourself struggling to maintain systems that worked effectively for years, forgetting routine tasks, or feeling overwhelmed by normal workload complexity.

Social interaction aversion develops as workplace relationships begin feeling more draining than supportive. Conversations with colleagues you previously enjoyed become effortful performances. Team meetings that once felt manageable start creating anxiety days in advance. Your natural need for social recovery time increases significantly.

Performance inconsistency patterns emerge as your work quality becomes unpredictable despite consistent effort. Some days you perform at your usual high standards while others feel impossible despite similar energy investment. This inconsistency often signals that your baseline energy reserves are depleting.

Physical symptom emergence includes headaches, muscle tension, digestive issues, and sleep disturbances that correlate with work stress rather than external health factors. These symptoms often represent your nervous system's response to chronic overwhelm rather than separate medical conditions.

Recovery Strategies That Don't Derail Your Career

Professional burnout recovery requires balancing necessary rest with career protection strategies that maintain your professional reputation and advancement opportunities. Strategic recovery approaches help you restore neurological function while preserving the career progress you've worked to achieve.

Systematic energy audit helps you identify specific activities, environments, and interactions that deplete your resources most significantly. This analysis guides targeted modifications that provide maximum recovery benefit without requiring complete work cessation or major career disruption.

Accommodation intensification involves temporarily increasing your workplace supports during recovery periods. This might include additional environmental modifications, schedule adjustments, or communication preferences that provide extra recovery space while maintaining work engagement.

Professional communication strategies help you explain necessary changes without revealing vulnerability that could affect career advancement. Frame recovery accommodations as productivity optimization rather than health problems, focusing on performance improvement rather than burnout management.

Sarah, a 36-year-old marketing director, managed her burnout recovery by requesting a temporary reduction in client meetings and additional project planning time. She presented these changes as process improvements that would enhance campaign quality, maintaining her professional reputation while providing necessary recovery space.

Work restructuring approaches identify which job responsibilities provide energy versus those that deplete resources. Temporary or permanent task redistribution can provide recovery opportunities while ensuring that critical work continues effectively.

Recovery timeline management helps you plan realistic timelines for neurological restoration while meeting professional obligations. Burnout recovery typically requires weeks or months rather than days, but this process can occur while maintaining career engagement through strategic modifications.

Support system activation involves leveraging professional relationships, mentors, and colleagues who can provide coverage, guidance, or advocacy during recovery periods.

These relationships often prove essential for maintaining career momentum while addressing health needs.

Building Burnout Prevention into Your Work Life

Sustainable career success requires systematic burnout prevention rather than crisis recovery management. Proactive approaches help you maintain optimal performance while preventing the energy depletion that leads to burnout episodes.

Energy management systematization creates structured approaches to allocating your limited resources across work demands while maintaining necessary reserves for unexpected challenges. This involves scheduling high-energy tasks during peak periods and protecting recovery time throughout workdays and weeks.

Masking reduction strategies identify opportunities to reduce the performance energy required for professional success. Every reduction in unnecessary masking preserves energy for actual work performance and career advancement activities.

Environmental optimization addresses workplace factors that create ongoing stress and energy drain. Systematic environmental improvements often provide immediate relief while supporting long-term sustainability and performance quality.

David, a 43-year-old financial analyst, prevented recurring burnout by implementing systematic environmental modifications including noise-canceling headphones, adjusted lighting, and structured meeting schedules that reduced daily energy drain by an estimated 30% while improving his analytical output quality.

Routine systematization provides predictable structure that reduces decision fatigue and cognitive load throughout workdays. Established routines for task management, communication, and energy allocation create efficiency that preserves resources for important work activities.

Social interaction budgeting helps you allocate social energy strategically across professional relationships and activities that support career advancement while maintaining necessary recovery periods. This systematic approach prevents social overwhelm while building valuable professional connections.

Regular monitoring protocols provide early detection systems that identify energy depletion before it reaches burnout levels. Systematic self-assessment helps you adjust workload, accommodation needs, or recovery activities before problems become critical.

When to Take Medical Leave and How to Return

Medical leave decisions require careful consideration of health needs, career implications, and legal protections that support both recovery and professional advancement. Strategic approaches help you access necessary time while protecting your career interests and return opportunities.

Leave necessity assessment involves evaluating signs that indicate recovery requires time away from work rather than workplace modifications. Severe executive function decline, physical health impacts, or inability to maintain basic professional performance might indicate that leave is necessary for effective recovery.

Legal protection research helps you understand Family and Medical Leave Act (FMLA) protections, Americans with

Disabilities Act accommodations, and organizational policies that support medical leave while protecting your job security and advancement opportunities (5).

Documentation preparation ensures that you have medical records and professional assessments that support leave requests while establishing the foundation for accommodation needs during return-to-work transitions.

Lisa, a 38-year-old operations manager, worked with her healthcare provider to document how autistic burnout was affecting her executive function and sensory processing, providing the medical foundation for FMLA leave that protected her position while allowing necessary recovery time.

Communication strategy development helps you explain leave needs to supervisors and HR representatives in ways that maintain professional credibility while securing necessary support. Focus on health management rather than crisis response, positioning leave as proactive wellness rather than emergency intervention.

Return-to-work planning begins during leave periods to ensure smooth transitions that maintain recovery progress while reestablishing professional effectiveness. This planning includes accommodation updates, workload adjustments, and communication strategies that support sustainable reintegration.

Recovery sustainability involves implementing systematic changes that prevent future burnout episodes rather than simply returning to previous work patterns. Use leave time to develop more effective energy management, accommodation strategies, and professional boundary setting.

Action Items: Burnout Prevention Protocol

This systematic approach helps you develop personalized burnout prevention strategies while creating early intervention protocols that protect both your health and career advancement.

Burnout Risk Assessment and Monitoring

1. **Personal Burnout Warning Sign Identification**
   Document your specific early warning indicators:

Physical Warning Signs Documentation

- Track headaches, muscle tension, sleep disturbances, or digestive issues that correlate with work stress
- Monitor energy levels throughout workdays and weeks to identify depletion patterns
- Note changes in sensory sensitivity that might indicate nervous system overload
- Document physical symptoms that appear during high-stress work periods

Cognitive and Emotional Indicators

- Monitor executive function changes including organization difficulties, memory problems, or decision-making challenges
- Track mood changes, irritability increases, or emotional numbness that correlate with work demands

- Note motivation declines, job satisfaction decreases, or work engagement reduction patterns
- Document social interaction tolerance changes and relationship strain development

Performance Pattern Monitoring

- Track work quality inconsistencies that might indicate energy depletion
- Monitor task completion times and efficiency changes over time
- Note increasing difficulty with routine tasks that previously felt manageable
- Document productivity fluctuations that don't correlate with workload changes

2. **Energy Expenditure Analysis** Understand how different work activities affect your energy reserves:

High-Energy Activity Identification

- List work activities that require significant mental or social energy
- Track masking demands throughout typical workdays
- Monitor sensory processing loads in different work environments
- Document social interaction costs and recovery requirements

Energy Recovery Assessment

- Identify activities, environments, or time periods that restore your energy

- Track how much recovery time you need after high-energy work activities

- Monitor weekend and vacation recovery patterns and effectiveness

- Document environmental or schedule modifications that improve energy management

Prevention Strategy Development

3. **Systematic Burnout Prevention Framework** Create proactive approaches that maintain sustainable work performance:

Daily Energy Management Protocol

- Design daily routines that balance energy expenditure with recovery opportunities

- Plan high-energy tasks during optimal performance periods

- Schedule recovery breaks between demanding activities

- Create end-of-day routines that provide closure and transition support

Weekly and Monthly Sustainability Planning

- Plan weekly schedules that include adequate recovery time

- Design monthly workload management that prevents energy accumulation

- Schedule regular accommodation effectiveness reviews and adjustments

- Plan vacation and time-off usage that provides genuine nervous system recovery

4. **Environmental and Accommodation Optimization** Implement workplace modifications that reduce ongoing energy drain:

Workspace Environment Enhancement

- Optimize lighting, sound, and temperature control within your workspace

- Implement sensory management tools that reduce environmental stress

- Create organizational systems that minimize cognitive load and decision fatigue

- Design workspace layouts that support your optimal work patterns

Communication and Social Interaction Management

- Establish email and meeting preferences that support your communication strengths

- Plan social interaction schedules that provide adequate recovery time

- Create professional boundary systems that protect your energy while maintaining relationships

- Develop networking and relationship building approaches that align with your social energy capacity

Early Intervention and Recovery Protocols

5. **Burnout Early Intervention System** Create systematic responses to warning signs that prevent crisis development:

Warning Sign Response Framework

- Develop specific interventions for each early warning sign you've identified
- Create escalation protocols that increase intervention intensity based on warning sign severity
- Plan communication strategies for requesting additional support during high-stress periods
- Design temporary accommodation requests that provide relief during challenging times

Crisis Prevention Planning

- Identify circumstances that would indicate need for medical leave or professional support
- Create documentation systems that track burnout symptoms and intervention effectiveness
- Plan support system activation protocols for times when you need additional assistance

- Develop communication strategies for supervisors and colleagues during burnout prevention periods

6. **Recovery and Return-to-Work Planning** Prepare systematic approaches for managing recovery if burnout occurs:

Medical Leave Preparation

- Research legal protections and organizational policies related to medical leave

- Prepare documentation that supports leave requests and accommodation needs

- Plan communication strategies that maintain professional relationships during absence

- Create return-to-work preparation protocols that ensure sustainable reintegration

Sustainable Return Strategies

- Design gradual reintegration approaches that prevent immediate re-burnout

- Plan accommodation updates that address factors contributing to original burnout

- Create ongoing monitoring systems that prevent future burnout episodes

- Develop professional development strategies that build on recovery insights and self-awareness

Professional Resilience Through Systematic Self-Care

Burnout prevention becomes a professional skill that enhances career sustainability while maintaining high performance standards. This systematic approach to energy management often produces better work outcomes while protecting your long-term health and career advancement opportunities.

Performance sustainability improves when energy management becomes as systematic as project management or technical skill development. Your proactive approach to burnout prevention often attracts professional recognition while creating work patterns that other colleagues eventually adopt.

Professional credibility grows when your systematic approach to health management demonstrates self-awareness and strategic thinking that transfers to other business challenges. Your burnout prevention expertise positions you as a resource for organizational wellness initiatives and team management effectiveness.

Career advancement often accelerates when sustainable work practices enable consistent high performance over extended periods rather than cycles of excellence followed by exhaustion and recovery.

The Foundation for Long-Term Professional Success

Your mastery of burnout prevention creates the foundation for sustainable career advancement that maintains your well-being while achieving professional objectives. This systematic approach to energy management provides competitive advantages that support rather than compromise your autism strengths.

Energy optimization enables performance consistency that builds professional reputation while protecting the neurological resources necessary for continued innovation and analytical excellence. Your systematic approach to sustainability often produces insights that benefit entire organizations.

Professional authenticity emerges when you can maintain high performance without the masking that contributes to burnout. This authenticity often attracts career opportunities that value your systematic thinking and analytical capabilities rather than requiring social performance.

Essential Elements for Burnout Prevention

- Early warning sign recognition enables intervention before energy depletion reaches crisis levels that require extended recovery

- Systematic energy management prevents the cumulative overload that leads to autistic burnout while maintaining professional effectiveness

- Strategic accommodation implementation addresses environmental and social factors that create ongoing neurological stress

- Proactive recovery planning provides structured approaches to restoration that protect career advancement while supporting health needs

- Professional communication strategies frame burnout prevention as performance optimization rather than health management

Your burnout prevention mastery provides the foundation for building professional support networks that accelerate career advancement while providing the understanding and assistance necessary for long-term autism-friendly professional success.

Chapter 14: Creating Your Professional Support Network

The promotion opportunity seemed perfect until Rebecca read the fine print: extensive travel, client entertainment, and team management responsibilities that would stretch her autism-related challenges beyond her current coping strategies. Instead of declining immediately, she reached out to her carefully cultivated professional network—three mentors who understood autism, five colleagues in similar roles, and two executive coaches with neurodiversity expertise. Within a week, she had specific strategies for managing each challenge and accepted the position that advanced her career by five years.

Professional success for autistic individuals rarely happens in isolation. Strategic support network development provides the guidance, advocacy, and practical assistance that accelerate career advancement while providing the understanding and accommodation support that traditional professional relationships often lack.

Finding Mentors Who Understand Autism

Traditional mentorship advice assumes that successful professionals can guide you by sharing their neurotypical career strategies. Autism-informed mentorship requires finding advisors who understand how your neurological differences affect professional development while providing guidance that leverages rather than minimizes your authentic strengths.

Autism-informed mentor identification involves finding professionals who demonstrate understanding of neurodiversity through their management style, public statements, or professional development approaches. These mentors might be openly autistic themselves, have autistic family members, or demonstrate neurodiversity support through their leadership practices.

Industry-specific autism mentorship connects you with professionals who understand both your field's requirements and autism's professional implications. A mentor in technology might provide different insights than one in healthcare or finance, because industry cultures vary significantly in their autism compatibility and advancement opportunities.

Systematic mentor research helps you identify potential mentors through professional organizations, conference speakers, LinkedIn profiles, or published articles that demonstrate autism awareness or neurodiversity advocacy. This research-based approach often produces better mentor relationships than random networking attempts.

Consider David, a 42-year-old engineering manager who identified his mentor through autism professional organizations rather than traditional industry networking. His mentor's understanding of autism workplace challenges provided guidance that helped David advance to director level while maintaining his authentic communication style and systematic work approach.

Value proposition development helps you approach potential mentors with clear understanding of what you can offer in exchange for guidance. Your systematic thinking, analytical capabilities, or specialized expertise often provide value that makes mentorship relationships mutually beneficial rather than one-sided requests for assistance.

Mentorship goal setting ensures that mentor relationships focus on specific professional development objectives rather than general career advice. Clear goals help mentors provide targeted guidance while demonstrating your commitment to implementing their suggestions and making progress toward advancement objectives.

Long-term relationship maintenance uses your natural reliability and systematic communication to build mentorship relationships that provide ongoing support throughout your career development rather than single consultation interactions.

Building Relationships with Other Autistic Professionals

Professional relationships with other autistic individuals provide unique benefits including shared understanding of workplace challenges, validation of autism experiences, and practical strategies that work specifically for neurodivergent professionals. These relationships often become essential career resources that provide support unavailable through traditional professional networking.

Autistic professional community identification involves finding colleagues who are open about their autism diagnosis or those who demonstrate neurodivergent characteristics in their professional approach. Online communities, professional organizations, and neurodiversity employee resource groups often provide initial connection opportunities.

Experience sharing frameworks help you build relationships based on mutual learning rather than simple social interaction. Share specific strategies that work for your autism-related challenges while learning from others' approaches to similar professional situations.

Career advancement collaboration enables group problem-solving approaches to professional challenges that individual efforts might not solve effectively. Multiple perspectives on autism workplace issues often produce innovative solutions that benefit all participants while advancing individual career objectives.

Sarah, a 35-year-old marketing analyst, joined an online group of autistic marketing professionals who shared strategies for handling client presentations, managing sensory challenges during conferences, and building professional relationships that honored their authentic communication styles. The group's collective wisdom helped her advance to director level while maintaining her autism accommodations.

Advocacy partnership allows collaborative efforts to improve workplace conditions, advance neurodiversity initiatives, or provide testimony for organizational policy changes that benefit all autistic employees. These partnerships often produce systemic improvements while building individual professional recognition.

Skill sharing networks connect autistic professionals with complementary expertise areas, creating informal consulting relationships that provide mutual professional development and business advancement opportunities.

Crisis support systems offer understanding and practical assistance during difficult professional periods when autism-related challenges temporarily affect career performance or workplace relationships.

Working with Coaches and Career Counselors

Professional coaching and career counseling can provide structured support for autism-specific career development when practitioners understand neurodiversity and can adapt their approaches to autism strengths and challenges. Strategic selection and utilization of these professional services accelerate career advancement while providing ongoing guidance.

Neurodiversity-informed practitioner selection involves researching coaches and counselors who demonstrate specific autism understanding rather than general disability awareness. Look for practitioners with autism training, neurodivergent clients, or published expertise in autism workplace issues.

Coaching goal alignment ensures that professional development focuses on leveraging autism strengths rather than overcoming neurodivergent characteristics. Effective autism coaching builds on systematic thinking, analytical capabilities, and attention to detail rather than trying to develop neurotypical social skills.

Career assessment adaptation uses autism-informed evaluation tools that account for different communication styles, social preferences, and work environment needs rather than standard assessments designed for neurotypical career patterns.

Jennifer, a 37-year-old operations director, worked with a coach who specialized in autism professional development to identify career advancement strategies that built on her systematic project management approach while providing support for networking and leadership challenges that felt unnatural but were necessary for senior roles.

Accommodation strategy development involves collaborative planning for workplace modifications, disclosure decisions, and communication approaches that support career advancement while honoring autism needs and preferences.

Interview and networking skill development adapts traditional career advancement techniques to autism processing styles and communication preferences, providing practical strategies that showcase professional capabilities without requiring masking or inauthentic performance.

Long-term career planning creates systematic approaches to professional development that account for autism energy management, burnout prevention, and accommodation needs while pursuing ambitious career advancement objectives.

Leveraging Employee Resource Groups

Employee Resource Groups (ERGs) focused on neurodiversity, disability, or inclusion provide structured opportunities for professional development, advocacy, and networking within your organization while building visibility and advancement opportunities that traditional performance alone might not provide.

ERG participation strategy involves contributing your autism expertise and systematic thinking to group initiatives while building professional relationships and organizational visibility that support career advancement objectives.

Leadership development opportunities within ERGs often provide experience with project management, event planning, and team coordination that builds leadership skills while contributing to causes that align with your personal values and professional interests.

Organizational influence building through ERG participation creates opportunities to affect policies, procedures, and cultural changes that benefit all neurodivergent employees while positioning you as a thought leader and change agent within your organization.

Michael, a 40-year-old financial analyst, leveraged his company's disability ERG to lead a neurodiversity education initiative that provided autism awareness training for managers while building his reputation as an expert in inclusive workplace practices. This visibility led to promotion opportunities and consulting requests from other organizational units.

Cross-functional networking through ERG activities provides access to professionals in different departments and organizational levels who might become valuable career contacts, collaboration partners, or advancement advocates.

Professional development programming offered through ERGs often includes training, speakers, and resources specifically relevant to neurodivergent career advancement that complement traditional professional development opportunities.

Advocacy skill development through ERG participation builds communication and influence capabilities that support both organizational change efforts and individual career advancement through improved professional relationship building and leadership experience.

Action Items: Support Network Mapping

This systematic approach helps you identify, develop, and maintain professional relationships that provide career advancement support while understanding and accommodating your autism-related needs and preferences.

Current Network Assessment and Gap Analysis

1. **Existing Relationship Evaluation** Analyze your current professional support systems:

Mentor and Advisor Assessment

- List current professional mentors and evaluate their autism understanding and support

- Assess whether existing advisors provide guidance that builds on vs. minimizes your autism strengths

- Document gaps in mentorship areas including industry expertise, autism awareness, or career level experience

- Evaluate relationship quality and mutual benefit in current mentorship arrangements

Professional Peer Network Analysis

- Identify colleagues who understand and support your autism-related needs and approaches

- Assess representation of autistic or neurodivergent professionals in your current network

- Document professional relationships that provide mutual learning and career advancement support

- Evaluate network diversity across industries, career levels, and organizational types

Professional Service Provider Evaluation

- Review coaches, counselors, or consultants you've used and their autism competency

- Assess whether professional development services account for autism strengths and challenges

- Identify gaps in professional support services that understand neurodiversity

- Evaluate cost-effectiveness and career impact of professional development investments

2. **Support Network Gap Identification** Determine specific relationship and resource needs:

Career Development Support Gaps

- Identify areas where autism-informed guidance would accelerate your professional advancement

- Document career challenges that would benefit from neurodiversity-aware mentorship or coaching

- Assess networking needs that require autism understanding for effective relationship building

- Evaluate advocacy needs for workplace accommodations or organizational culture change

Industry and Functional Expertise Needs

- Identify industry contacts who could provide autism-informed career guidance

- Document functional expertise areas where autism perspective would benefit your development

- Assess leadership development needs that account for autism leadership strengths and challenges

- Evaluate entrepreneurship or alternative career path guidance needs

Strategic Network Development Planning

3. **Mentor and Advisor Acquisition Strategy** Develop systematic approaches to building mentorship relationships:

Autism-Informed Mentor Identification Framework

- Research potential mentors through autism professional organizations and conferences

- Identify industry leaders who demonstrate neurodiversity support through public statements or policies

- Connect with autism professionals through LinkedIn, professional associations, or published articles
- Seek introductions through existing autism-aware contacts or ERG connections

Mentorship Relationship Development Protocol

- Prepare value propositions that demonstrate what you can offer potential mentors
- Develop systematic approaches to mentor outreach that respect their time while demonstrating serious commitment
- Create mentorship goal frameworks that focus discussions on specific career advancement objectives
- Plan relationship maintenance systems that provide ongoing value while receiving guidance

4. **Peer Network Building Strategy** Create connections with other autistic and neurodivergent professionals:

Professional Community Engagement Planning

- Identify autism professional organizations, online communities, and local meetup groups
- Plan conference attendance that focuses on neurodiversity professional development sessions
- Develop strategies for contributing expertise to autism professional communities

- Create systems for maintaining relationships with autism colleagues across different organizations

Cross-Industry Network Development

- Connect with autistic professionals in complementary industries or functional areas
- Build relationships with autism advocates and thought leaders who could provide career guidance
- Develop partnerships with other autism professionals for collaboration and mutual support
- Create accountability partnerships that support career advancement goals and autism accommodation strategies

Support System Utilization and Maintenance

5. **Professional Development Service Integration**
   Access and utilize autism-informed professional services effectively:

Coaching and Counseling Strategy Development

- Research and select autism-competent coaches or career counselors based on specific development needs
- Develop coaching goals that leverage autism strengths while addressing career advancement challenges

- Plan coaching relationships that provide ongoing support rather than crisis intervention
- Create systems for implementing coaching guidance while maintaining authentic professional approaches

ERG and Organizational Resource Utilization

- Participate strategically in neurodiversity or disability employee resource groups
- Contribute autism expertise to organizational inclusion initiatives and policy development
- Seek leadership opportunities within ERGs that build management experience and organizational visibility
- Leverage ERG connections for career advancement opportunities and professional development

6. **Network Maintenance and Growth Strategy** Sustain and expand professional relationships systematically:

Relationship Maintenance Protocol

- Create systems for regular communication with mentors, peers, and professional service providers
- Develop approaches for providing value to network contacts while receiving career support

- Plan annual relationship reviews that assess effectiveness and identify improvement opportunities
- Create succession planning for mentor relationships as your career progresses

Network Impact Assessment and Optimization

- Monitor how professional relationships contribute to career advancement and autism support
- Evaluate return on investment for professional development services and network participation
- Adjust network composition based on changing career objectives and development needs
- Share successful network strategies with other autism professionals to build community support

Professional Advancement Through Strategic Relationships

Your support network success multiplies when relationships are built on mutual value and authentic understanding rather than simple career advancement requests. Autism-informed professional relationships often provide more effective career support than traditional networking because they address the specific challenges and leverage the unique strengths that affect neurodivergent professional development.

Community building around autism professional success creates opportunities for collaborative advancement that benefits multiple careers while advancing neurodiversity awareness and accommodation within various industries and organizations.

Expertise development in autism professional issues positions you as a valuable resource within your support network while building recognition that can advance your career through speaking, writing, and consulting opportunities.

Advocacy integration with career advancement creates professional development that benefits both individual success and systemic change for autism workplace inclusion and support.

The Strategic Framework for Professional Support

Your professional support network becomes most effective when it reflects the systematic, research-based approach that characterizes autism strengths. Strategic relationship building often produces better career outcomes than broad networking while requiring less social energy and providing more authentic professional development.

Professional authenticity in relationship building attracts contacts who value your systematic thinking and analytical capabilities rather than expecting neurotypical social performance. These authentic relationships often provide more effective long-term career support.

Mutual benefit focus ensures that professional relationships provide value to all participants rather than one-sided support requests. Your autism strengths often enable you to contribute unique insights and assistance that make relationships rewarding for all involved parties.

Strategic Support Development Principles

- Autism-informed mentorship provides career guidance that builds on neurodivergent strengths rather than attempting to overcome neurological differences

- Professional relationships with other autistic individuals offer unique understanding and practical strategies unavailable through traditional networking

- Specialized coaching and counseling services accelerate career development when practitioners understand autism workplace implications

- Employee resource group participation creates organizational visibility while advancing neurodiversity initiatives that benefit all participants

- Systematic network development produces more effective professional relationships than random networking while requiring less social energy

Your professional support network provides the foundation for exploring alternative career paths that may offer greater autism compatibility and professional satisfaction than traditional employment structures.

Chapter 15: Alternative Career Paths and Entrepreneurship

The resignation letter sat on Marcus's laptop for two weeks before he finally clicked send. After eight years as a senior software engineer at a prestigious technology company, he was walking away from a six-figure salary, comprehensive benefits, and clear advancement opportunities to start his own consulting practice. His colleagues thought he was crazy. His autism diagnosis six months earlier had helped him understand that traditional employment, no matter how successful, might never provide the environmental control and authentic work relationships he needed for long-term sustainability.

Eighteen months later, Marcus was earning 40% more than his corporate salary while working with clients who valued his systematic approach to complex problems. His home office provided perfect sensory control, his schedule accommodated his natural energy patterns, and his direct communication style had become a business asset rather than an accommodation need.

Consulting and Freelancing Considerations

Independent consulting and freelancing offer autism-friendly alternatives to traditional employment by providing greater control over work environment, client relationships, and project selection. However, successful self-employment requires careful evaluation of both autism-related advantages and challenges that affect business sustainability.

Environmental control benefits represent one of the strongest advantages of independent work. You can design workspace environments that optimize your sensory needs, eliminate open office distractions, and create the organizational systems that support your optimal performance without requiring accommodations or justifications to employers.

Client relationship management differs significantly from employee relationships because consulting arrangements focus on deliverable outcomes rather than social integration or cultural fit. Your direct communication style and systematic project approach often become business advantages when clients value results over relationship maintenance.

Schedule flexibility advantages allow you to structure work around your natural energy patterns, accommodation needs, and optimal performance periods. You can schedule demanding analytical work during peak cognitive hours while handling administrative tasks during lower-energy periods.

Consider Sarah, a 36-year-old marketing consultant who left corporate marketing to start her own practice. Her autism-driven attention to detail and systematic campaign analysis attracted clients who needed thorough market research and data-driven strategy development. Her ability to work during optimal hours improved her analytical quality while eliminating the energy drain of daily office social interaction.

Revenue variability challenges require systematic financial planning and business development that account for irregular income patterns. Your systematic thinking strengths support effective financial management, but successful consulting requires tolerance for income uncertainty that might create stress if not managed strategically.

Business development requirements involve marketing, networking, and client acquisition activities that might challenge autism social and communication preferences. However, expertise-based marketing often aligns better with autism strengths than relationship-based business development approaches.

Administrative complexity includes invoicing, tax management, insurance acquisition, and legal compliance that require systematic attention to detail. Your natural organization capabilities often make business administration manageable, but these responsibilities represent additional workload beyond client-focused activities.

Starting Autism-Friendly Businesses

Entrepreneurship enables you to create organizations that naturally support autism strengths while providing products or services that benefit from your systematic thinking and analytical capabilities. Successful autism-friendly businesses often address market needs that neurotypical approaches overlook or handle inadequately.

Systematic problem-solving businesses leverage your natural analytical thinking to address complex challenges that require thorough research, detailed analysis, and methodical solution development. These businesses might include data analysis services, process optimization consulting, or research-based advisory services.

Quality-focused service businesses build on your attention to detail and commitment to excellence in areas where thoroughness creates significant client value. Examples include technical writing, financial analysis, software testing, or compliance auditing services that benefit from meticulous attention to accuracy and completeness.

Technology and automation businesses often align naturally with autism strengths because they emphasize logical systems, clear cause-and-effect relationships, and systematic problem-solving approaches. Software development, database design, or automation consulting businesses frequently succeed when led by autistic entrepreneurs.

David, a 41-year-old database consultant, started a business helping small companies optimize their data systems after recognizing that most generic solutions failed to address specific organizational needs. His systematic approach to database analysis and autism-driven attention to data integrity attracted clients who needed thorough solutions rather than quick fixes.

Niche expertise businesses develop around specialized knowledge areas where your systematic learning style and pattern recognition create significant expertise depth. These businesses might focus on specific industries, technical areas, or problem types where your analytical capabilities provide clear competitive advantages.

Business model considerations affect how well entrepreneurship aligns with your autism characteristics and professional objectives. Service businesses require ongoing client interaction while product businesses might enable more independent work patterns. Subscription models provide revenue predictability while project-based work offers schedule flexibility.

Scaling strategy planning involves determining how business growth aligns with your autism accommodation needs and energy management requirements. Some autistic entrepreneurs thrive by building teams while others prefer maintaining small, personally manageable operations.

Remote Work Optimization

Remote work environments often provide autism-friendly alternatives to traditional office settings while maintaining employment benefits and career advancement opportunities. Strategic remote work optimization can transform challenging jobs into sustainable career paths that leverage your strengths.

Sensory environment control enables you to create workspace conditions that optimize your performance without requiring employer accommodations. Home offices allow lighting, sound, and temperature adjustments that might be impossible in shared workplace environments.

Social interaction management through remote work provides natural boundaries around workplace social demands while maintaining professional relationships through structured communication channels. Video meetings, email correspondence, and project collaboration can occur without the energy drain of constant interpersonal navigation.

Schedule optimization within remote work arrangements often allows greater flexibility around your natural energy patterns, accommodation needs, and optimal work periods. Many remote positions provide more autonomy over daily schedules than traditional office-based roles.

Jennifer, a 37-year-old project manager, negotiated full remote work arrangements that transformed her job satisfaction and performance. Working from her controlled home environment eliminated sensory overwhelm while structured virtual team meetings actually improved her communication effectiveness compared to chaotic in-person gatherings.

Communication preference accommodation becomes easier in remote work environments where written communication often predominates over verbal interaction. Your systematic communication style and thorough documentation practices often become business advantages in remote team environments.

Productivity measurement focus in remote work arrangements typically emphasizes deliverable outcomes rather than time spent in office or social participation. This outcome-based evaluation often favors autism strengths in systematic work completion and quality delivery.

Technology optimization for remote work success involves selecting tools and systems that support your organizational needs and communication preferences. Your systematic approach to technology evaluation often produces more effective remote work setups than colleagues who focus primarily on convenience factors.

Portfolio Career Strategies

Portfolio careers combine multiple income sources through various projects, clients, or part-time positions that collectively provide financial stability while offering diversity and flexibility that traditional single-employer careers might not accommodate. This approach can provide autism-friendly alternatives while maintaining professional growth and financial security.

Income diversification strategies reduce dependence on single employers while providing flexibility to adjust work composition based on changing autism needs, energy levels, or life circumstances. Multiple income streams can include consulting projects, part-time employment, training delivery, or product sales.

Skill combination approaches leverage your systematic thinking across different professional areas or industries, creating unique value propositions that single-focus careers might not provide. Your analytical capabilities might apply to financial analysis, process improvement, technical writing, and strategic planning across various organizations.

Energy management benefits of portfolio careers enable you to balance high-energy client work with lower-demand activities,creating sustainable work patterns that prevent burnout while maintaining professional engagement. You can alternate between intensive analytical projects and routine administrative tasks based on your daily energy capacity.

Consider Lisa, a 38-year-old operations specialist who developed a portfolio career including part-time process improvement consulting, technical writing projects, and teaching business analysis courses. This combination provided income stability while allowing her to focus on different types of work based on her energy levels and autism accommodation needs.

Client relationship variety in portfolio careers provides multiple professional relationships without the intensive social demands of single workplace cultures. You can work with clients who appreciate your direct communication style while avoiding those who require extensive relationship management or social performance.

Professional development acceleration often occurs through portfolio careers because exposure to different organizations, industries, and challenges provides broader learning opportunities than single-employer advancement paths. Your systematic learning approach benefits from this variety while building expertise across multiple areas.

Risk management considerations involve ensuring that portfolio income sources provide adequate financial stability while maintaining professional reputation across multiple relationships. Your systematic approach to planning and organization supports effective portfolio management when applied strategically.

Market positioning strategies help you develop professional reputation that attracts diverse opportunities while maintaining consistent quality and service delivery across different portfolio components. Your autism strengths in reliability and systematic work completion often become valuable differentiators in competitive markets.

Action Items: Alternative Path Evaluation

This systematic assessment helps you evaluate non-traditional career paths and determine which alternatives might provide better autism compatibility while supporting your professional and financial objectives.

Current Career Satisfaction and Constraint Analysis

1. **Traditional Employment Assessment** Evaluate your current employment situation and autism compatibility:

Workplace Challenge Documentation

- List specific aspects of traditional employment that create ongoing stress or energy drain

- Document accommodation needs that are difficult to obtain or maintain in employer environments

- Assess social and sensory challenges that affect your performance in typical workplace settings

- Evaluate how organizational politics, cultural expectations, or management styles conflict with your autism traits

Career Advancement Limitation Analysis

- Identify ways that traditional career paths might limit your advancement due to autism-related factors

- Document requirements for advancement (networking, social performance, travel) that conflict with your needs

- Assess whether your autism strengths are recognized and valued in current organizational culture

- Evaluate long-term sustainability of masking and accommodation energy costs in traditional employment

Financial and Benefit Dependency Assessment

- Calculate your actual dependency on employer-provided benefits and steady income

- Assess your financial preparation for variable income or self-employment transition

- Evaluate insurance, retirement, and other benefit needs that alternative careers must address

- Document minimum income requirements for sustainable life management and autism support needs

2. **Alternative Career Interest and Aptitude Evaluation** Assess your suitability and interest in different non-traditional career paths:

Entrepreneurship and Business Ownership Assessment

- Evaluate your interest in business development, client acquisition, and revenue generation activities

- Assess your tolerance for financial uncertainty and business risk management

- Document business ideas that could leverage your autism strengths and specialized expertise

- Evaluate your capacity for business administration, marketing, and customer relationship management

Consulting and Freelancing Capability Analysis

- Identify expertise areas where you could provide valuable independent consulting services

- Assess your ability to market services and build client relationships that support sustainable business

- Evaluate your capacity for project management, deadline adherence, and quality delivery without employer oversight

- Document potential consulting markets and competitive analysis for your specialized skills

Market Research and Opportunity Assessment

3. **Industry and Market Analysis for Alternative Careers** Research opportunities that align with your autism strengths and career objectives:

Consulting Market Research

- Identify potential consulting opportunities in your expertise areas and target industries

- Research market rates, demand patterns, and competitive factors for your specialized skills

- Analyze client needs that your autism strengths (systematic thinking, attention to detail) could address effectively

- Evaluate market trends that might create new opportunities for autism-informed consulting services

Remote Work and Freelance Opportunity Analysis

- o Research companies and industries that support remote work arrangements and independent contractors

- o Identify platforms, networks, and job boards that specialize in remote and freelance opportunities

- o Assess which of your skills transfer effectively to remote work environments and freelance project structures

- o Evaluate remote work trends in your industry and their potential for long-term career sustainability

4. **Financial Planning and Risk Assessment** Develop realistic financial planning for alternative career transitions:

Transition Financial Planning

- o Calculate savings needed to support alternative career transitions and variable income periods

- o Plan for business startup costs, equipment needs, and professional development investments

- o Develop emergency fund requirements that account for irregular income and business development periods

- Create financial timelines for alternative career transitions that minimize risk while enabling change

Revenue and Business Model Planning

- Project realistic income potential for different alternative career options based on market research

- Develop business models that align with your autism accommodation needs and energy management requirements

- Plan pricing strategies that reflect your expertise value while remaining competitive in target markets

- Create revenue diversification strategies that provide income stability while building alternative career momentum

Implementation and Transition Strategy Development

5. **Alternative Career Transition Planning** Create systematic approaches to transitioning from traditional employment to alternative career paths:

Gradual Transition Strategy Development

- Plan part-time or project-based work that builds alternative career experience while maintaining current income

- Develop professional reputation and client relationships before complete traditional employment departure

- Create skill development plans that prepare you for independent work challenges and opportunities
- Design transition timelines that minimize financial risk while enabling authentic career development

Professional Infrastructure Development

- Plan business setup requirements including legal structure, insurance, and financial management systems
- Develop marketing materials, professional websites, and networking strategies that attract target clients
- Create operational systems for project management, client communication, and quality delivery
- Plan professional development and continuing education that maintains expertise and market relevance

6. **Success Measurement and Optimization Planning** Develop metrics and adjustment strategies for alternative career success:

Performance and Satisfaction Monitoring

- Create measurement systems for financial success, professional satisfaction, and autism accommodation effectiveness

- Plan regular assessment of alternative career alignment with your values, goals, and autism needs

- Develop feedback collection systems from clients or customers that guide service improvement and professional development

- Design adjustment protocols for modifying alternative career approaches based on experience and changing needs

Long-Term Development and Growth Planning

- Plan professional development strategies that build expertise and market position in alternative career paths

- Create networking and relationship building approaches that support alternative career advancement

- Develop strategies for scaling alternative careers while maintaining autism accommodation needs and energy management

- Plan legacy building and mentorship opportunities that share alternative career success with other autism professionals

Professional Freedom Through Alternative Paths

Alternative career paths often provide the environmental control and authentic relationship patterns that enable autism strengths to flourish while eliminating many traditional workplace challenges. Success in these paths typically requires systematic planning and gradual transition rather than impulsive career changes.

Professional authenticity increases in alternative careers where your systematic approach and direct communication become business assets rather than accommodation needs. Clients and customers often value the thoroughness and reliability that autism traits provide.

Market differentiation emerges when your autism strengths create unique value propositions that distinguish your services from conventional approaches. Your attention to detail, analytical thinking, and systematic problem-solving often address market needs that neurotypical providers overlook.

Sustainable success in alternative careers builds on working with your autism traits rather than against them, creating professional patterns that maintain your energy while producing excellent outcomes for clients and customers.

The Strategic Foundation for Career Innovation

Your systematic approach to evaluating alternative career paths often produces more thorough analysis than conventional career change decisions. This analytical foundation increases success probability while ensuring that career transitions align with both professional objectives and autism accommodation needs.

Risk management through systematic planning enables alternative career transitions that maintain financial stability while pursuing professional authenticity and environmental compatibility.

Professional development continues through alternative careers with greater alignment between learning activities and your natural interests and learning styles.

Alternative Career Success Principles

- Environmental control and authentic relationships in alternative careers often support autism strengths better than traditional employment

- Systematic business planning and gradual transitions reduce risks while building alternative career success

- Market differentiation through autism strengths creates competitive advantages in consulting, entrepreneurship, and freelancing

- Remote work optimization provides autism-friendly employment alternatives while maintaining traditional career benefits

- Portfolio career strategies combine multiple income sources while offering flexibility and variety that prevent burnout

Your mastery of alternative career evaluation provides the foundation for creating a personalized professional development plan that builds on your authentic strengths while achieving your career and life objectives.

Broader Perspectives

Recognition that traditional employment represents only one career option marks a significant shift from accommodating limitations to optimizing opportunities. Alternative career paths often provide better autism compatibility while offering professional growth that honors your authentic strengths and accommodation needs.

The systematic evaluation of these alternatives provides data for informed decision-making that considers both immediate needs and long-term professional objectives. Your analytical approach to career planning often produces insights that benefit other autism professionals considering similar transitions.

Success in alternative career paths creates opportunities to model autism-friendly professional approaches while building businesses and services that may specifically benefit other neurodivergent individuals seeking similar career solutions.

Conclusion: Your Ongoing Professional Evolution

The conference room had changed, but not in any way that others would notice. The same fluorescent lights hummed overhead, the same beige walls reflected the familiar corporate aesthetic, and the same quarterly reports demanded attention from the assembled management team. But for Rachel, everything was different. Two years after her autism diagnosis at age 37, she sat at that conference table not as someone trying to fit in, but as someone who understood exactly how her brain worked and why that was a professional asset.

As the senior director of operations, Rachel no longer apologized for her systematic approach to complex problems. She didn't mask her need for written follow-ups after verbal discussions. She had stopped forcing herself to enjoy team-building activities that drained her energy. Instead, she had learned to position her autism traits as the analytical strengths and reliable consistency that had earned her three promotions in eighteen months.

Your professional evolution continues beyond this book, building on the foundation of self-understanding and strategic career development that transforms autism from accommodation need to competitive advantage.

Creating Your Personalized Career Development Plan

Sustainable professional success requires ongoing development that honors your autism traits while pursuing ambitious career objectives. Your personalized plan integrates the strategies you've learned into systematic approaches that guide long-term professional growth and satisfaction.

Authentic strength development focuses your professional growth on capabilities that align with your autism traits rather than trying to overcome neurological differences. Your systematic thinking, analytical capabilities, and attention to detail become the foundation for advanced skills that accelerate career advancement.

Environmental optimization planning ensures that your work environments continue supporting your optimal performance as your roles and responsibilities change. This includes anticipating accommodation needs for leadership positions, travel requirements, or organizational changes that might affect your workplace compatibility.

Career trajectory customization aligns advancement opportunities with your autism strengths while developing strategies for managing challenges that senior roles might present. Your leadership development builds on authentic capabilities rather than neurotypical performance expectations.

Energy management systematization creates sustainable approaches to professional growth that prevent burnout while maintaining high performance standards. Your understanding of autism energy patterns guides workload management, project selection, and professional development timing.

Professional relationship evolution builds on your networking and communication strategies to create ongoing relationships that support career advancement while providing autism understanding and accommodation support.

Resources for Continued Growth

Professional development for autistic individuals benefits from resources that understand neurodiversity while providing advanced career guidance. These specialized resources complement traditional professional development with autism-informed perspectives and practical strategies.

Autism professional organizations provide ongoing education, networking opportunities, and advocacy resources that support career advancement while advancing autism workplace understanding. Organizations like the Autistic Self Advocacy Network and Autism @ Work initiatives offer continuing education and community support (6).

Neurodiversity-focused conferences combine professional development with autism-specific career strategies, providing learning opportunities that traditional professional conferences might not address. These events often feature successful autistic professionals sharing advanced strategies for career growth and workplace success.

Specialized coaching and mentoring with autism-informed practitioners provides ongoing guidance for complex career challenges and advanced professional development that builds on your neurodivergent strengths.

Industry-specific autism networks connect you with professionals in your field who understand both industry requirements and autism workplace implications. These networks provide ongoing learning and advancement opportunities that general autism resources might not address.

Research and publication opportunities in autism workplace topics position you as a thought leader while contributing to knowledge that benefits other professionals. Writing, speaking, and consulting on autism career topics often become valuable professional development activities.

Building on Your Success

Professional achievement creates opportunities for advanced career development that leverages your growing expertise in autism-informed workplace success. Your success becomes a foundation for helping other professionals while advancing your own career objectives.

Leadership development builds on your systematic thinking and reliable performance to create management approaches that benefit from autism traits. Your understanding of accommodation needs and inclusion practices often makes you an effective leader for diverse teams.

Mentorship opportunities emerge as other autistic professionals seek guidance from someone who has successfully navigated career advancement while maintaining authentic self-expression. Your mentoring expertise becomes a valuable professional skill while contributing to autism community development.

Organizational consulting leverages your understanding of autism workplace needs to help employers develop more effective neurodiversity initiatives. This expertise often creates career advancement opportunities while improving workplace conditions for other autistic employees.

Industry innovation results when your different perspective and systematic problem-solving approach produce solutions that conventional thinking overlooked. These innovations often position you for senior roles while demonstrating the business value of neurodiversity.

Professional legacy building involves creating lasting improvements in autism workplace acceptance and accommodation that benefit future professionals while establishing your reputation as a leader in neurodiversity advancement.

Paying It Forward to Other Late-Diagnosed Professionals

Your career success creates opportunities and responsibilities to support other autistic professionals who are beginning their own journey toward authentic professional development. This support strengthens the entire autism professional community while building your reputation as a leader and advocate.

Mentorship provision offers other late-diagnosed professionals the guidance and understanding that you might have needed during your own career development. Your systematic approach to mentoring often produces effective guidance relationships that benefit both parties.

Workplace advocacy involves using your professional position and credibility to advance autism accommodation and inclusion within your organization. Your success demonstrates the business value of autism inclusion while creating better conditions for current and future autistic employees.

Knowledge sharing through writing, speaking, or training helps other professionals learn from your experience while positioning you as an expert in autism workplace success. These activities often create professional development opportunities while contributing to autism community advancement.

Resource development involves creating tools, frameworks, or resources that help other autistic professionals navigate career challenges more effectively. Your systematic thinking often produces practical resources that benefit multiple professionals.

Community building strengthens professional networks that support autism career advancement while providing you with ongoing relationships that continue supporting your own professional growth.

The Continuous Journey

Your professional evolution doesn't end with career success—it continues as you refine your understanding of how autism affects your work while pursuing increasingly ambitious professional objectives. This ongoing development creates opportunities for continued growth while building expertise that benefits others.

Self-awareness deepening continues as you gain more experience working authentically in professional environments. Each new role or challenge provides additional data about your strengths, accommodation needs, and optimal working conditions.

Strategy refinement improves your approaches to workplace success as you test different techniques and learn from various professional experiences. Your systematic learning style supports continuous improvement in autism-informed career strategies.

Impact expansion grows as your professional success creates opportunities to influence larger systems, mentor more professionals, and contribute to autism workplace research and advocacy at organizational and industry levels.

The conference room where Rachel sits today represents not just her individual success, but the growing recognition that autism brings distinctive value to professional environments. Her journey from accommodation-seeking employee to confident leader exemplifies the career transformation possible when autism traits are understood as professional assets rather than limitations to overcome.

Your professional evolution continues with each authentic conversation, each successfully managed challenge, and each opportunity to demonstrate that autism-informed approaches often produce superior results while requiring less energy than masking-based performance.

The systematic thinking that helped you navigate this career guide will continue serving you as you build a professional life that honors your authentic self while achieving the career success you've always been capable of reaching. Your autism isn't something to overcome—it's the foundation for a distinctive professional approach that creates value for you, your colleagues, and the organizations fortunate enough to benefit from your systematic excellence.

Professional Transformation Success

Your career transformation from late autism diagnosis to professional authenticity creates a template that other professionals can follow while establishing you as a leader in autism workplace advancement. This success demonstrates that autism-informed career strategies often produce better outcomes than conventional approaches while requiring less energy and creating more sustainable professional satisfaction.

The strategies you've learned and implemented become increasingly sophisticated as you gain experience applying them to new challenges and opportunities. Your growing expertise in autism-friendly professional development positions you for continued advancement while contributing to positive change in workplace culture and inclusion practices.

Your professional future builds on this foundation of self-understanding and strategic career management, creating opportunities for continued growth that aligns with your authentic strengths while achieving ambitious career objectives that seemed impossible before you understood how your autism could become your greatest professional asset.

Appendix A: Templates and Worksheets

The stack of papers on Jessica's desk told the story of her professional transformation. Accommodation request letters with approval stamps, performance review notes highlighting her systematic thinking as a business asset, and networking conversation templates that had helped her build relationships without exhausting small talk. Each document represented a milestone in her journey from hiding her autism to leveraging it as a professional strength.

These templates and worksheets provide the practical tools you need to implement the strategies discussed throughout this guide. They're designed to save you time while ensuring your communications are professional, clear, and effective in achieving your autism-related workplace goals.

Disclosure Conversation Scripts

Professional disclosure conversations require careful preparation to ensure you communicate your needs clearly while positioning your autism as a professional asset. These scripts provide frameworks you can adapt to your specific situation and communication style.

Initial Disclosure to Direct Supervisor Script

"I wanted to schedule time to discuss some workplace accommodations that would help me maintain my high performance level and take on additional responsibilities. I've recently been diagnosed with autism spectrum disorder, which explains some of the work patterns and preferences you may have noticed. This diagnosis helps me understand why I work so effectively with clear processes and structured environments.

I'm requesting a few specific modifications that will allow me to continue contributing effectively to our team goals. These accommodations include [specific list of 2-3 key needs]. I have medical documentation to support this request, and I believe these changes will actually improve my productivity and the quality of my work output.

I want to emphasize that this diagnosis doesn't change my commitment to excellence or my ability to perform my job duties. In fact, understanding my autism helps me work more efficiently and leverage my strengths in systematic thinking and attention to detail. I'm happy to discuss how we can implement these accommodations in a way that supports both my needs and our department objectives."

Follow-up Disclosure Discussion Script

"I wanted to check in about how the accommodations are working and whether you've noticed any impact on my productivity or team contributions. Since implementing [specific accommodations], I've been able to [specific performance improvements or achievements].

I'm committed to making sure these arrangements continue to benefit both my performance and our team effectiveness. If you have any concerns or suggestions for adjustments, I'm happy to discuss modifications that ensure we're meeting both my needs and our business objectives. I also want to make sure my colleagues understand that these accommodations help me work at my best, which ultimately benefits our entire team's success."

Accommodation Modification Request Script

"I'd like to discuss modifying one of my current accommodations based on how it's working in practice. The [specific accommodation] has been helpful, but I think [specific modification] would be even more effective for [specific business outcome]. This adjustment would help me [specific performance benefit] while maintaining the collaborative approach that's important to our team.

I've researched the implementation requirements and believe this modification would be straightforward to implement. Could we explore this adjustment? I'm confident it will improve both my effectiveness and my contribution to our team objectives."

Team Communication Script for Accommodation Disclosure

"I wanted to let you know that I'll be using [specific accommodation] going forward. This change will help me maintain my focus and productivity while contributing to our team projects. You might notice [specific visible changes], but this shouldn't affect our collaboration or communication.

If you have any questions about how we can work together effectively, please let me know. I'm committed to maintaining the quality of our teamwork while using tools that help me perform at my best. I appreciate your understanding and support as I implement these changes."

Accommodation Request Letters

Formal accommodation requests require specific language and structure to ensure legal compliance while positioning your needs as productivity enhancements rather than special requirements.

Comprehensive Accommodation Request Letter Template

[Date]

[Supervisor Name] [Title] [Department] [Company Name]

Dear [Supervisor Name],

I am formally requesting workplace accommodations under the Americans with Disabilities Act to optimize my performance in my role as [job title]. I have been diagnosed with Autism Spectrum Disorder by [licensed professional], which affects my sensory processing, communication style, and work environment needs.

Medical Condition Impact: My autism affects my workplace performance in the following areas:

- Sensory processing requires environmental modifications for optimal concentration

- Communication preferences favor written formats and structured meetings for effective collaboration

- Executive function benefits from clear priorities and systematic work organization

Requested Accommodations:

1. **Environmental Modifications**
   - Noise-canceling headphones for concentration during analytical work
   - Desk lamp to reduce dependence on fluorescent lighting

- Workspace positioning away from high-traffic areas

2. **Communication Accommodations**
   - Written meeting summaries and advance agendas when possible
   - Email for non-urgent communication to allow processing time
   - Structured check-ins rather than impromptu discussions for project updates

3. **Schedule and Routine Support**
   - Consistent work schedule when possible to support optimal performance patterns
   - Advance notice for schedule changes when feasible
   - Brief breaks between meetings for processing and preparation time

Business Benefits: These accommodations will enable me to:

- Maintain the high-quality analytical work that has earned consistent positive feedback
- Increase productivity by reducing environmental distractions and communication inefficiencies
- Continue contributing my systematic thinking and attention to detail to team projects
- Take on additional responsibilities that leverage my strengths in [specific areas]

Implementation Support: I am committed to working collaboratively with you and HR to implement these accommodations effectively. I can provide additional information about specific products or arrangements, and I'm flexible about implementation details that serve both my needs and our business objectives.

I have attached medical documentation supporting this request and am available to discuss implementation timelines and any questions you may have. Thank you for your consideration and support.

Sincerely, [Your name] [Your contact information]

Attachment: Medical documentation from [provider name and credentials]

Accommodation Request Follow-up Letter Template

[Date]

[HR Representative Name] [Human Resources Department] [Company Name]

Dear [HR Representative Name],

I am following up on my accommodation request submitted on [date] regarding workplace modifications for my autism spectrum disorder diagnosis. I wanted to provide additional information and check on the status of my request.

Additional Implementation Details: After further consideration, I can provide the following specifics about accommodation implementation:

- [Specific accommodation]: Estimated cost of [amount] with implementation timeline of [timeframe]

- [Specific accommodation]: No cost modification requiring [specific changes]

- [Specific accommodation]: [Implementation details and alternatives if needed]

Performance Impact Data: Since submitting my initial request, I have documented the following performance patterns that support the business case for these accommodations:

- [Specific productivity data or performance metrics]

- [Quality improvements or efficiency gains when accommodation needs are met]

- [Collaboration effectiveness when communication preferences are accommodated]

Next Steps: I am ready to begin the interactive process to finalize accommodation details and implementation timelines. I'm available for meetings, can provide additional documentation if needed, and am committed to ensuring these accommodations support both my optimal performance and our team effectiveness.

Please let me know what additional information would be helpful and what our next steps should be for implementing these accommodations.

Thank you for your attention to this request.

Best regards, [Your name] [Your contact information]

Performance Review Preparation Guides

Performance reviews provide opportunities to demonstrate how your autism traits contribute to business success while addressing any accommodation needs or professional development goals.

Pre-Review Self-Assessment Framework

Accomplishment Documentation:

1. List specific achievements and their business impact
   - Project completions with quality metrics
   - Process improvements you initiated or implemented
   - Problems you solved using systematic thinking
   - Recognition or feedback received from colleagues or clients

2. Autism Strength Contribution Analysis
   - How attention to detail prevented errors or improved quality
   - Systematic thinking applications that benefited team or organizational goals
   - Reliability examples that supported project success or team stability
   - Innovation resulting from different perspective or analytical approach

3. Professional Development Progress
   - Skills developed that build on autism strengths
   - Training completed that enhanced systematic thinking or analytical capabilities

- Accommodation effectiveness and any needed adjustments
- Leadership or mentoring contributions related to inclusion or process improvement

Performance Review Discussion Outline

Opening Statement: "I want to review my contributions this year and discuss how my systematic approach and attention to detail have supported our team objectives. I'm also interested in exploring opportunities for additional responsibilities that leverage these strengths."

Achievement Presentation:

- Present specific accomplishments with quantified business impact
- Connect achievements to autism-related strengths without over-explaining
- Demonstrate consistent performance and reliable delivery
- Show innovation or improvement resulting from systematic thinking

Professional Development Discussion:

- Request development opportunities that build on analytical and systematic strengths
- Discuss accommodation effectiveness and any needed adjustments
- Propose leadership or project opportunities that utilize autism advantages

- Address any performance feedback with specific improvement plans

Goal Setting Framework:

- Set goals that leverage systematic thinking and analytical capabilities

- Request projects that benefit from attention to detail and process orientation

- Plan professional development that aligns with autism learning styles

- Establish metrics that reflect autism-friendly performance indicators

Networking Conversation Starters

Professional networking conversations require preparation to feel natural while gathering useful information and building meaningful relationships. These conversation frameworks help you network effectively while honoring your communication style.

Industry Conference Conversation Templates

Speaker Approach Framework: "I really appreciated your presentation on [specific topic]. Your point about [specific detail] relates directly to work I'm doing on [your relevant project]. I'm particularly interested in [specific aspect] because my systematic approach to [related area] has shown [specific results or insights]. Could you recommend resources for learning more about [specific subtopic]?"

Vendor/Exhibitor Conversation Template: "I'm researching solutions for [specific business challenge] and noticed your [product/service] addresses [relevant capability]. In my experience with [related systems/processes], the key factors for success are [specific criteria]. How does your solution handle [specific requirement] and what implementation support do you provide for [specific consideration]?"

Peer Professional Networking Script: "I'm [your name] from [company], working in [your function]. I noticed you're also in [their field/function] - I'm curious about your experience with [specific industry challenge or trend]. In my work, I've found that [your systematic approach/insight] produces [specific results]. What approaches have worked well for you in addressing [related challenge]?"

Professional Development Focused Conversations

Career Advancement Discussion Framework: "I'm working on developing expertise in [specific area] and noticed your background includes [relevant experience]. I'm particularly interested in how [specific skill/knowledge area] applies to [business challenge]. My analytical approach to [related work] has shown [specific results], and I'm exploring how to expand this into [advancement area]. What advice would you have for someone developing expertise in this field?"

Mentorship Request Conversation: "I've been following your work in [specific area] and particularly admire your approach to [relevant challenge]. I'm [your role] with [background summary] and have found success using systematic thinking for [specific applications]. I'm interested in developing [specific skill/area] and would value guidance from someone with your experience. Would you be open to periodic conversations about [specific development goals]?"

Collaboration Opportunity Discussion: "Your presentation on [topic] highlighted some interesting parallels with my work on [related project]. My systematic analysis of [relevant area] has produced [specific insights/results] that might complement your work on [their project area]. Would you be interested in exploring how our different approaches might benefit both our projects?"

Professional Interest and Learning Conversations

Industry Expertise Gathering Framework: "I'm researching [specific topic/trend] and your experience with [relevant area] would provide helpful perspective. In my analysis of [related subject], I've noticed [specific pattern/trend] that seems to connect with [their expertise area]. What trends are you seeing in [specific aspect] and how do you think they'll affect [business application]?"

Process and System Discussion Template: "I noticed your company has implemented [specific system/process] that addresses [business challenge]. In my work optimizing [related processes], I've found that [systematic approach/insight] produces [specific benefits]. How has your implementation handled [specific consideration] and what lessons learned might apply to [related context]?"

Innovation and Problem-Solving Conversation: "Your approach to [specific challenge] is interesting because it addresses [business problem] differently than conventional methods. My systematic thinking about [related problem] has led me to [specific insights/approaches] that produce [results]. I'm curious how your different perspective on [problem area] developed and what results you're seeing."

Appendix B: Industry-Specific Considerations

The elevator pitch Michael had practiced sounded perfect until he realized that healthcare consulting required different autism considerations than his previous technology role. The systematic thinking that made him exceptional at software architecture needed different positioning when applied to hospital workflow optimization. Each industry creates unique opportunities and challenges for autistic professionals, requiring tailored approaches to maximize success.

Understanding how autism traits interact with specific industry cultures and requirements helps you make informed career decisions while developing strategies that leverage your strengths within particular professional contexts.

Technology and Engineering

Technology and engineering fields often provide autism-friendly environments because technical competence typically outweighs social performance in advancement decisions. These industries frequently value the systematic thinking, attention to detail, and analytical problem-solving that characterize autism strengths.

Cultural Advantages for Autistic Professionals

Technology cultures often embrace neurodiversity because different thinking styles drive innovation and problem-solving excellence. Many tech companies explicitly recruit autistic professionals through specialized programs that recognize autism traits as business assets rather than accommodation needs (7).

Engineering environments typically focus on measurable outcomes, systematic processes, and logical problem-solving approaches that align naturally with autism cognitive patterns. The emphasis on technical accuracy and detailed analysis creates professional contexts where autism traits become competitive advantages.

Remote work prevalence in technology provides environmental control that supports optimal performance while eliminating many traditional workplace challenges. Distributed teams often communicate primarily through written channels that favor autism communication strengths.

Career Advancement Strategies

Technical leadership roles often build on autism strengths in systematic thinking and attention to detail rather than requiring extensive social performance. Engineering management positions can leverage your ability to understand complex systems while developing processes that support team effectiveness.

Specialization opportunities in technology allow deep expertise development that aligns with autism learning patterns and interests. Becoming a subject matter expert in specific technologies or domains provides career advancement through technical excellence rather than broad relationship management.

Innovation and research roles often benefit from autism traits including pattern recognition, systematic analysis, and persistence with complex problems. Research and development positions typically provide environmental control while rewarding different thinking approaches.

Industry-Specific Challenges and Solutions

Agile methodologies common in technology can create challenges through frequent interruptions, rapid context switching, and intensive social interaction. However, modified agile approaches that include written communication, structured meetings, and clear role definitions often work well for autistic team members.

Open office environments prevalent in tech companies create sensory challenges that require accommodation strategies. Many technology companies readily approve environmental modifications because they understand the connection between optimal work environments and productivity.

Client interaction requirements in consulting or customer-facing roles might conflict with autism social preferences. However, technical consulting often emphasizes problem-solving expertise over relationship management, making client interaction more manageable.

Healthcare and Education

Healthcare and education industries offer opportunities for autistic professionals in analytical and systematic roles, though direct patient or student interaction positions might present social and sensory challenges that require careful consideration.

Autism-Compatible Healthcare Roles

Health informatics and data analysis positions leverage autism strengths in systematic thinking and attention to detail while focusing on analytical work rather than direct patient care. These roles often provide clear success metrics and structured work environments.

Research coordination and clinical trials management benefit from autism traits including attention to detail, systematic documentation, and process adherence. These positions require analytical thinking while providing structured environments with clear protocols.

Quality assurance and compliance roles in healthcare utilize autism strengths in systematic review and pattern recognition to ensure regulatory adherence and patient safety. These positions often provide clear guidelines and measurable outcomes.

Laboratory and diagnostic positions often align well with autism traits because they emphasize technical accuracy, systematic procedures, and analytical interpretation rather than extensive social interaction.

Education Sector Opportunities

Curriculum development and instructional design leverage autism strengths in systematic thinking and attention to detail while creating structured educational materials and programs. These roles often provide creative opportunities within systematic frameworks.

Educational technology and data analysis positions combine autism analytical strengths with education industry applications. These roles often focus on system optimization and performance measurement rather than direct teaching responsibilities.

Special education support, particularly autism-related services, can provide meaningful career opportunities for autistic professionals who understand autism firsthand while contributing to student success and system improvement.

Research and evaluation roles in education utilize autism systematic thinking for program assessment, outcome measurement, and process improvement within educational organizations.

Industry Considerations and Adaptations

Healthcare environments can present sensory challenges through medical equipment noise, bright lighting, and chemical odors that require accommodation planning. However, many healthcare organizations understand the importance of environmental modifications for optimal staff performance.

Patient and family interaction requirements in healthcare roles might conflict with autism social preferences. Roles that emphasize technical competence over bedside manner often provide better autism compatibility while still contributing to patient care.

Educational environments can create challenges through noise, social complexity, and schedule unpredictability. However, support roles and behind-the-scenes positions often provide autism-friendly alternatives while contributing to educational success.

Finance and Consulting

Finance and consulting industries value systematic thinking and analytical capabilities that align well with autism strengths, though client relationship management and business development activities might require accommodation strategies.

Finance Industry Autism Advantages

Analytical roles in finance directly utilize autism strengths in systematic thinking, pattern recognition, and attention to detail. Financial analysis, risk assessment, and compliance positions often provide clear success metrics and structured work environments.

Research and modeling positions benefit from autism persistence with complex problems and systematic approach to data analysis. These roles typically focus on technical accuracy rather than social performance while providing advancement opportunities.

Operations and process improvement roles leverage autism ability to identify inefficiencies and systematize workflows. Finance operations often appreciate systematic approaches to process optimization and quality control.

Regulatory compliance and audit positions utilize autism attention to detail and systematic review capabilities while providing clear guidelines and measurable outcomes.

Consulting Opportunities and Challenges

Specialized consulting in technical areas often aligns well with autism expertise development and systematic problem-solving approaches. Technical consulting emphasizes analytical competence over relationship management while providing variety and intellectual challenge.

Process improvement and operational consulting leverage autism strengths in systematic analysis and efficiency optimization. These consulting areas often focus on measurable outcomes rather than relationship building.

Client relationship management in consulting can present challenges for autistic professionals but can be managed through structured communication approaches and focus on expertise demonstration rather than social performance.

Business development requirements in consulting might conflict with autism social preferences but can be addressed through systematic approaches to networking and expertise-based marketing strategies.

Professional Development Strategies

Certification and credential development in finance often align with autism learning patterns and provide clear advancement pathways based on technical competence rather than social networking.

Specialization strategies allow deep expertise development that provides competitive advantages while building on autism learning strengths and analytical capabilities.

Leadership development in finance and consulting can build on autism systematic thinking and reliable performance while addressing communication and team management challenges through structured approaches.

Creative Industries

Creative industries present unique opportunities and challenges for autistic professionals, with success often depending on finding roles that balance creative expression with systematic approaches to project management and quality control.

Autism Strengths in Creative Fields

Technical production roles in creative industries often utilize autism attention to detail and systematic thinking while contributing to creative projects. Video editing, audio engineering, and production management positions provide structured approaches to creative work.

Design and development positions that emphasize systematic thinking alongside creativity can provide excellent opportunities for autistic professionals. User experience design, web development, and graphic design roles often benefit from autism analytical thinking.

Writing and content development leverage autism research skills and systematic thinking while providing creative expression opportunities. Technical writing, content strategy, and editorial positions often align well with autism communication strengths.

Quality control and project management roles in creative industries utilize autism organizational strengths while ensuring creative projects meet specifications and deadlines.

Industry Adaptation Strategies

Creative collaboration requirements can be managed through structured brainstorming approaches, written communication protocols, and clear role definitions that honor both creative process and autism working style.

Client presentation and feedback sessions in creative industries might require accommodation strategies but can be managed through systematic preparation and focus on project outcomes rather than interpersonal dynamics.

Freelance and contract opportunities in creative fields often provide environmental control and project variety while building on autism creative and analytical strengths.

Professional Development Approaches

Portfolio development strategies can showcase autism systematic approach to creative work while demonstrating consistent quality and reliable delivery.

Networking in creative industries can focus on expertise demonstration and project collaboration rather than social relationship building.

Business development for creative professionals can utilize systematic approaches to client acquisition and project management while building on creative and analytical strengths.

Government and Nonprofit

Government and nonprofit sectors often provide structured environments, clear policies, and mission-driven work that can align well with autism values and working styles while offering stability and advancement opportunities.

Government Sector Opportunities

Policy analysis and research positions in government utilize autism systematic thinking and analytical capabilities while contributing to public service and policy development.

Regulatory compliance and oversight roles leverage autism attention to detail and systematic review capabilities while providing clear guidelines and public service opportunities.

Data analysis and program evaluation positions in government often provide structured work environments while utilizing autism analytical strengths for public benefit.

Administrative and operational roles in government can provide stability and clear advancement pathways while utilizing autism organizational and systematic thinking strengths.

Nonprofit Sector Advantages

Program evaluation and outcome measurement roles in nonprofits utilize autism analytical thinking while contributing to mission-driven organizations and social impact.

Grant writing and fundraising positions can leverage autism research skills and systematic thinking while supporting organizational sustainability and program development.

Operations and administration roles in nonprofits often provide structured environments while contributing to meaningful causes and community impact.

Advocacy and policy work in autism-related nonprofits can provide career opportunities that utilize personal experience while contributing to community support and systems change.

Sector-Specific Considerations

Government environments often provide strong accommodation support and clear policies while offering job security and structured advancement opportunities.

Nonprofit work can provide meaningful career opportunities but might require salary considerations and resource limitations that affect accommodation availability.

Public service roles often emphasize competence and systematic thinking over social networking while providing opportunities for community contribution and systems improvement.

Appendix C: Resources and References

The bookmark folder titled "Career Resources" on Amanda's laptop contained forty-seven carefully researched links to autism professional development organizations, legal resources, and career counseling services. Each bookmark represented hours of systematic research to identify resources that actually understood autism rather than simply offering general disability guidance. Her organized approach to resource collection had accelerated her career development while helping three colleagues find similar support.

Professional success requires ongoing access to autism-informed resources that provide guidance, legal protection, and community support throughout your career development. These resources offer specialized assistance that general professional development services often cannot provide.

Autism Organizations and Support Groups

National and international autism organizations provide professional development resources, networking opportunities, and advocacy support specifically designed for autistic adults in professional settings.

National Autism Organizations

The Autistic Self Advocacy Network (ASAN) provides policy advocacy, professional development resources, and community support focused on autistic adult needs and workplace rights. ASAN offers toolkits for workplace advocacy and accommodation while promoting autism acceptance in professional settings (8).

Autism Speaks' workplace initiatives include employer education programs and professional development resources, though their medical model approach may not align with all autistic professionals' perspectives. Their Autism at Work program connects autistic professionals with participating employers.

The Autism Society of America offers local chapter support, professional development workshops, and advocacy resources for autistic adults. Local chapters often provide networking opportunities and peer support specific to regional employment markets.

Autism Women & Nonbinary Network (AWN) addresses the specific needs of autistic women and nonbinary individuals in professional settings, offering resources that address gender-specific workplace challenges and career development strategies.

Professional Autism Networks

LinkedIn autism professional groups provide networking opportunities, job postings, and career advice specifically for autistic professionals. These groups offer peer support and industry-specific guidance from professionals with autism experience.

Industry-specific autism professional organizations exist in technology, healthcare, education, and other fields, providing targeted career development resources and networking opportunities within specific professional contexts.

Local autism professional meetups and support groups offer in-person networking and career development opportunities. Many metropolitan areas host regular autism professional gatherings that provide community support and local resource sharing.

International Autism Professional Resources

Autism advocacy organizations in Canada, United Kingdom, Australia, and other countries provide professional development resources that may offer different perspectives and approaches to autism workplace success.

International autism conferences often include professional development tracks and networking opportunities that provide global perspectives on autism career advancement and workplace accommodation.

Career Counseling Resources

Autism-informed career counseling requires practitioners who understand both professional development and autism workplace implications. These specialized services provide guidance that general career counseling might not address.

Autism-Specialized Career Counselors

Licensed professional counselors with autism specialization provide career assessment, development planning, and transition support specifically designed for autistic professionals. Look for practitioners with autism training and experience rather than general disability counseling.

Vocational rehabilitation counselors in some states offer autism-specific services including career assessment, job search support, and accommodation assistance. State vocational rehabilitation agencies often provide free or low-cost services for eligible individuals.

Private practice career coaches with autism expertise offer specialized services including interview preparation, accommodation planning, and career transition support. Research practitioners' autism credentials and client testimonials before engaging services.

Autism-Informed Assessment Tools

Career assessment instruments designed for autistic individuals account for different communication styles, processing patterns, and work preferences that standard assessments might not capture accurately.

Autism-specific interest inventories help identify career paths that align with autism traits and learning patterns rather than forcing conventional career categories that might not fit autistic strengths.

Accommodation assessment tools help identify specific workplace modifications that would optimize performance while providing documentation for accommodation requests.

Professional Development Services

Autism-informed professional development workshops focus on leveraging autism strengths rather than overcoming neurodivergent characteristics. These services often address communication, leadership, and career advancement from autism perspectives.

Interview coaching services with autism specialization provide preparation that accounts for autism communication patterns while helping professionals present their capabilities effectively.

Workplace integration coaching helps autistic professionals navigate new job environments, implement accommodations, and build professional relationships that honor autism communication and social preferences.

Legal Resources for Workplace Rights

Understanding and enforcing workplace rights requires access to legal resources that specialize in disability law and autism workplace issues. These resources provide both education and advocacy support for professional protection.

Disability Rights Organizations

The Disability Rights Education & Defense Fund (DREDF) provides legal advocacy, policy development, and educational resources for disability rights enforcement including autism workplace accommodations and anti-discrimination protection.

National Disability Rights Network (NDRN) offers state-by-state legal advocacy services and resources for disability rights enforcement. State Protection & Advocacy agencies provide free legal assistance for eligible individuals facing workplace discrimination.

Equal Employment Opportunity Commission (EEOC) provides information about ADA workplace rights, discrimination filing procedures, and employer obligations regarding autism accommodations. EEOC offers both educational resources and enforcement assistance (9).

Legal Aid and Advocacy Services

Disability law clinics at law schools often provide free or low-cost legal assistance for autism workplace issues while training future attorneys in disability rights law.

Private practice disability attorneys specialize in workplace discrimination and accommodation cases. Look for attorneys with autism experience and successful accommodation track records.

Bar association disability law sections in many states provide attorney referrals and legal resources specific to disability rights and workplace accommodation law.

Self-Advocacy Legal Resources

Autism self-advocacy legal guides provide step-by-step information for enforcing workplace rights, filing accommodation requests, and responding to discrimination without requiring attorney assistance.

Legal aid websites offer template documents, filing procedures, and legal information specific to autism workplace rights and accommodation enforcement.

Workplace rights workshops specifically for autistic individuals provide legal education and self-advocacy training that addresses autism-specific workplace challenges and rights enforcement.

Recommended Reading and Research

Autism professional development benefits from resources that combine current research with practical career guidance specifically designed for autistic adults in professional settings.

Autism Career Development Books

"Developing Talents" by Temple Grandin provides career guidance that emphasizes building on autism strengths rather than overcoming deficits. Grandin's work offers practical advice from autism perspective with specific industry recommendations.

"The Complete Guide to Asperger's Syndrome" by Tony Attwood includes workplace and career sections that address autism professional challenges and strategies from clinical and practical perspectives.

"Been There. Done That. Try This!" edited by Tony Attwood offers practical strategies from autistic adults including workplace and career advice based on lived experience rather than clinical theory.

Research Publications and Journals

Autism research journals including "Autism," "Journal of Autism and Developmental Disorders," and "Autism in Adulthood" publish workplace and employment research that provides evidence-based information about autism career success factors.

Harvard Business Review articles on neurodiversity in the workplace provide business perspective on autism professional strengths and organizational benefits of autism inclusion.

Academic research on autism employment outcomes, accommodation effectiveness, and career development provides evidence-based information for advocacy and accommodation planning.

Professional Development Publications

Industry publications that address neurodiversity and autism in professional settings provide current information about best practices, legal developments, and successful autism inclusion initiatives.

Autism advocacy publications often include career and workplace sections that provide practical guidance and community perspectives on professional development and workplace success.

Business publications increasingly address neurodiversity as competitive advantage, providing organizational perspective that can inform autism professionals about market trends and employer attitudes.

Online Resources and Websites

Autism professional development websites offer ongoing resources including job boards, accommodation guides, and career advice specifically for autistic professionals.

Neurodiversity advocacy websites provide current information about workplace rights, accommodation strategies, and professional development opportunities for autistic individuals.

Professional association websites in various industries increasingly include neurodiversity resources and autism-specific guidance for career development within specific fields.

Appendix D: Emergency Protocols

The meltdown began in the quarterly budget meeting when three simultaneous crises—unexpected client changes, server failures, and a fire alarm test—overwhelmed Kevin's ability to process information systematically. Fifteen minutes later, he was hyperventilating in the stairwell, unable to think clearly or communicate effectively. Without an emergency protocol, Kevin's professional reputation could have suffered permanent damage. With systematic crisis management strategies, he returned to work the next day with colleagues who understood and respected his need for structured recovery.

Professional emergencies require immediate response strategies that protect both your well-being and career interests while providing clear steps for crisis management and recovery.

Workplace Crisis Management

Autism-related workplace crises often develop rapidly from sensory overload, unexpected changes, or overwhelming social demands. Having predetermined response protocols prevents crisis escalation while maintaining professional relationships and protecting career advancement.

Immediate Crisis Recognition and Response

Early warning sign identification helps you recognize crisis development before complete overwhelm occurs. These signs might include increased heart rate, difficulty processing information, heightened sensory sensitivity, or feeling trapped in social situations.

Immediate exit strategies provide predetermined methods for leaving overwhelming situations professionally. These might include bathroom breaks, brief outdoor walks, or requesting brief postponement of meetings for "urgent calls" or "document review."

Safe space identification in your workplace includes quiet areas where you can decompress privately. Know locations of empty conference rooms, outdoor spaces, stairwells, or storage areas where you can recover without public observation.

Professional Communication During Crisis

Crisis communication scripts provide prepared language for explaining temporary absence without detailed disclosure. Examples include "I need to step out for a brief call," "I need to review some documents," or "I'll be back in fifteen minutes."

Supervisor notification protocols help you communicate with management when crisis requires extended absence. Prepared messages can explain need for recovery time without compromising professional reputation.

Colleague explanation strategies provide simple language for team members who might be affected by your temporary absence. Focus on return timing rather than crisis details.

Crisis Prevention Integration

Environmental monitoring throughout workdays helps you identify accumulating stress before crisis levels develop. Regular self-assessment of sensory load, social demand, and energy levels enables early intervention.

Schedule modification strategies prevent crisis-inducing situations through advance planning. This includes spacing out demanding activities, building in recovery time, and identifying high-risk periods for increased vigilance.

Accommodation utilization ensures that existing workplace modifications are maximized to prevent crisis development. Regular assessment of accommodation effectiveness helps identify needed adjustments before problems become critical.

Meltdown Recovery Strategies

Autistic meltdowns require specific recovery approaches that restore neurological function while protecting professional relationships and career standing. Recovery strategies address both immediate needs and longer-term professional relationship management.

Immediate Recovery Protocols

Physical safety prioritization ensures that you're in a safe location where recovery can occur without additional stress or professional exposure. This might mean leaving your workspace temporarily or finding private space within your building.

Sensory regulation techniques help restore neurological function through systematic approaches to overwhelming stimulation. This might include noise-canceling headphones, removing yourself from bright lighting, or finding quiet spaces for decompression.

Breathing and grounding exercises provide systematic approaches to restoring calm and cognitive function. Simple techniques like box breathing or progressive muscle relaxation can be practiced quickly in private spaces.

Professional Recovery Management

Absence explanation strategies provide professional language for explaining temporary unavailability without detailed medical disclosure. Focus on return timing and work continuity rather than personal health details.

Work coverage protocols ensure that critical responsibilities are addressed during recovery periods. This might include notifying key colleagues, rescheduling meetings, or arranging temporary task coverage.

Return-to-work preparation helps you reintegrate professionally after crisis episodes. This includes reviewing what triggered the crisis and implementing prevention strategies for similar situations.

Long-term Relationship Management

Colleague education strategies help team members understand autism-related needs without compromising your professional reputation. Focus on work effectiveness rather than medical details when discussing accommodation needs.

Professional reputation protection ensures that crisis episodes don't damage career advancement opportunities. This includes demonstrating consistent high performance and reliable recovery patterns.

Accommodation adjustment protocols help you modify workplace supports based on crisis experiences. Use crisis data to identify needed environmental or schedule modifications that prevent similar episodes.

When to Involve HR or Legal Counsel

Some workplace situations require professional intervention to protect your rights and career interests. Understanding when to escalate issues ensures appropriate response while preserving professional relationships when possible.

HR Involvement Indicators

Accommodation denial or inadequate implementation that affects your ability to perform job duties requires HR intervention to ensure legal compliance and proper support provision.

Discrimination or harassment related to autism disclosure or accommodation use necessitates formal HR involvement to address policy violations and protect your workplace rights.

Manager resistance to accommodation implementation or retaliation for accommodation requests requires HR intervention to ensure proper accommodation provision and legal compliance.

Workplace safety concerns related to sensory overload or crisis management might require HR involvement to implement proper emergency protocols and support systems.

Legal Consultation Criteria

Formal discrimination complaints may require legal consultation to understand filing procedures, documentation requirements, and potential outcomes before proceeding with formal action.

Accommodation denials that appear to violate ADA requirements might benefit from legal review to determine whether formal complaints or legal action would be appropriate.

Retaliation for accommodation requests or autism disclosure might require legal consultation to understand protection options and appropriate response strategies.

Complex accommodation situations involving multiple departments or significant costs might benefit from legal review to ensure proper implementation and compliance.

Documentation Requirements

Incident documentation for HR or legal consultation should include dates, witnesses, specific language used, and impacts on work performance or career advancement.

Communication records including emails, meeting notes, and accommodation requests provide evidence for HR or legal review of workplace issues.

Medical documentation and accommodation needs assessment support formal complaints and legal consultation by establishing the basis for accommodation requirements.

Performance records demonstrating consistent work quality help support discrimination claims by showing that workplace issues aren't related to job performance deficiencies.

Self-Advocacy Scripts for Difficult Situations

Professional self-advocacy requires prepared language that protects your rights while maintaining collaborative relationships and professional credibility. These scripts provide frameworks for addressing challenging situations effectively.

Accommodation Resistance Scripts

"I understand there may be concerns about implementing this accommodation. I'd like to discuss how we can address any challenges while ensuring I can perform my job duties effectively. Could we explore alternative approaches that meet both my needs and organizational requirements?"

"The accommodation I've requested is necessary for me to perform my essential job functions effectively. I'm happy to provide additional documentation or discuss implementation alternatives, but I need this support to maintain my performance level."

"I want to work collaboratively to implement accommodations that support both my needs and our business objectives. Could we schedule time to discuss specific implementation concerns and identify solutions that work for everyone?"

Discrimination Response Scripts

"I'm concerned that my treatment may be related to my autism diagnosis rather than my work performance. I'd like to discuss this situation with you directly before involving HR. Could we schedule time to address my concerns and ensure fair treatment going forward?"

"I believe the decision to [specific action] may have been influenced by my autism accommodation requests rather than legitimate business reasons. I'd like to understand the rationale behind this decision and ensure it's not related to my disability status."

"I'm experiencing what appears to be retaliation for requesting accommodations. This concerns me both professionally and legally. I'd like to resolve this situation appropriately while protecting my rights and maintaining our working relationship."

Colleague Misunderstanding Scripts

"I appreciate your concern, but my [accommodation/behavior] is related to my autism and helps me work effectively. I understand it might seem unusual, but it allows me to contribute my best work to our team."

"I know my communication style might seem direct, but I want to clarify that I'm focused on getting the best results for our project. If my approach seems abrupt, please let me know how I can communicate more effectively while maintaining clarity."

"My need for [specific accommodation] isn't a preference— it's necessary for me to do my job effectively. I understand it might require some adjustment in how we work together, but I'm committed to making our collaboration successful."

Manager Conflict Resolution Scripts

"I'd like to discuss how my autism affects my work style and what that means for our team's success. I want to ensure you understand how my systematic approach and attention to detail contribute to our objectives."

"I sense there may be some misunderstanding about my accommodation needs. Could we schedule time to discuss how these modifications actually improve my productivity and benefit our team's results?"

"I want to address any concerns you might have about my performance or work style. I believe some issues might stem from misunderstanding about how autism affects my professional approach rather than actual performance problems."

Client or External Relationship Scripts

"I want to ensure our project communication is as effective as possible. I work best with written follow-ups and structured agendas, which actually helps ensure we cover all important points and maintain clear records."

"My systematic approach to [project area] means I ask detailed questions and want thorough documentation. This helps me deliver the high-quality results you're expecting and prevents misunderstandings later."

"I appreciate your patience with my communication style. My direct questions and systematic approach help me understand your needs clearly so I can provide the best possible service."

Crisis Prevention and Management Integration

Professional crisis management becomes most effective when integrated into daily work routines rather than treated as emergency response only. Systematic approaches to crisis prevention often eliminate the need for emergency protocols while building professional reputation for reliability and self-awareness.

Daily Monitoring Systems

Energy level tracking throughout workdays provides early warning data that helps prevent crisis development. Simple hourly self-assessment on a 1-10 scale identifies patterns and triggers before they become overwhelming.

Stress accumulation awareness helps you recognize when multiple smaller challenges are building toward crisis levels. Systematic tracking of meetings, deadlines, environmental factors, and social demands provides crisis prevention data.

Environmental condition monitoring including noise levels, lighting changes, and workspace disruptions helps you identify and address crisis triggers before they affect performance or well-being.

Professional Integration Strategies

Accommodation optimization ensures that existing workplace supports are utilized effectively to prevent crisis development. Regular review of accommodation effectiveness helps identify needed adjustments before problems become critical.

Schedule management protocols include building recovery time into demanding periods, spacing out high-energy activities, and identifying optimal timing for challenging tasks or interactions.

Communication system development helps colleagues understand your needs while maintaining professional relationships that support rather than hinder crisis prevention efforts.

Organizational Support Building

Supervisor education about autism workplace needs helps managers recognize and support crisis prevention while understanding that accommodation use demonstrates professional self-awareness rather than weakness or special treatment requests.

Team integration ensures that crisis prevention strategies enhance rather than disrupt collaborative work. Colleagues who understand autism workplace needs often become supportive allies rather than obstacles to effective crisis management.

Organizational culture development through autism advocacy and education creates environments where crisis prevention strategies are normalized rather than stigmatized, benefiting all employees while supporting autism inclusion.

Professional Growth Through Crisis Management

Effective crisis management often becomes a professional asset that demonstrates self-awareness, systematic thinking, and proactive problem-solving capabilities. Many successful autistic professionals report that their crisis management expertise eventually contributed to leadership opportunities and organizational consulting roles.

Skill Development Recognition

Crisis management expertise often translates to valuable professional skills including stress management, systematic problem-solving, and workplace safety awareness that benefit entire organizations.

Self-regulation capabilities developed through autism crisis management provide leadership advantages in high-pressure situations where emotional regulation and systematic thinking are essential.

Prevention planning skills developed for autism crisis management often apply to organizational risk management, project planning, and change management initiatives that advance career development.

Professional Reputation Building

Reliable recovery patterns demonstrate professional resilience that builds confidence among supervisors and colleagues about your ability to handle challenging situations effectively.

Crisis prevention expertise positions you as a resource for workplace wellness initiatives and stress management program development that can advance career opportunities.

Self-advocacy capabilities developed through crisis management often translate to valuable communication and negotiation skills that support career advancement and leadership development.

Tools for Professional Emergency Management

- Systematic crisis recognition prevents overwhelming situations from escalating while protecting professional relationships and career advancement

- Immediate response protocols provide professional methods for managing autism-related workplace emergencies without compromising career reputation

- Recovery strategies restore neurological function while maintaining work continuity and colleague relationships

- Professional self-advocacy scripts protect autism workplace rights while preserving collaborative relationships and advancement opportunities

- Crisis prevention integration creates sustainable work patterns that eliminate most emergency situations while building professional reputation for reliability

Your mastery of autism crisis management provides the foundation for sustainable professional success that transforms potential vulnerabilities into demonstrations of self-awareness and systematic thinking that often become career assets rather than accommodation needs.

Professional Resilience Through Systematic Support

Recognition that autism workplace challenges require systematic preparation and response strategies marks the difference between crisis management and crisis prevention. The tools and resources provided in these appendices transform potential workplace difficulties into manageable situations that often strengthen rather than compromise professional relationships and career advancement.

Your systematic approach to resource utilization, industry analysis, and crisis management creates a professional foundation that supports not just immediate success but long-term career growth that builds on authentic strengths while providing the support systems necessary for sustained professional excellence.

The templates, industry insights, resources, and emergency protocols become increasingly sophisticated as you gain experience applying them to various professional situations. This growing expertise in autism-informed workplace success positions you for continued advancement while contributing to positive change in organizational culture and professional inclusion practices.

References

(1) U.S. Equal Employment Opportunity Commission. (2021). *The Americans with Disabilities Act: A Guide to Disability Rights Laws*. Washington, DC: EEOC Publications.

(2) Job Accommodation Network. (2020). *Workplace Accommodations: Low Cost, High Impact*. Morgantown, WV: JAN Publications.

(3) Harvard Business Review. (2019). "Neurodiversity as a Competitive Advantage." *Harvard Business Review*, 97(3), 96-103.

(4) Austin, R. D., & Pisano, G. P. (2017). Neurodiversity as a competitive advantage. *Harvard Business Review*, 95(3), 96-103.

(5) U.S. Department of Labor. (2021). *Family and Medical Leave Act: Employee Rights and Responsibilities*. Washington, DC: DOL Publications.

(6) Autistic Self Advocacy Network. (2020). *Workplace Accommodations and Professional Development for Autistic Adults*. Washington, DC: ASAN Publications.

(7) Microsoft Corporation. (2021). *Autism Hiring Program: Creating Inclusive Workplaces Through Neurodiversity*. Redmond, WA: Microsoft Diversity & Inclusion Publications.

(8) Autistic Self Advocacy Network. (2022). *Professional Development and Career Advancement for Autistic Adults*. Washington, DC: ASAN Career Resources.

(9) U.S. Equal Employment Opportunity Commission. (2022). *Autism Spectrum Disorders in the Workplace: ADA*

Requirements and Best Practices. Washington, DC: EEOC Technical Assistance Publications.

www.ingramcontent.com/pod-product-compliance
Lightning Source LLC
Chambersburg PA
CBHW062200270326
41930CB00009B/1596